There's More to

Heart Health

than Cholesterol

There's More to

Heart

Health

than Cholesterol

Catherine Saxelby

**A 10-Step Plan
to Lower Your Cholesterol
and Protect Your Heart**

MARLOWE & COMPANY
NEW YORK

THERE'S MORE TO HEART HEALTH THAN CHOLESTEROL

Copyright © Catherine Saxelby 2001, 2002

Published by
Marlowe & Company
An Imprint of Avalon Publishing Group Incorporated
161 William Street, 16th Floor
New York, NY 10038

First published as *Nutrition for the Healthy Heart* by Hardie Grant Books
in Australia in 2001. This edition published by arrangement.

Library of Congress Cataloging-in-Publication Data

Saxelby, Catherine.
[Nutrition for the healthy heart]
There's more to heart health than cholesterol / by Catherine Saxelby.
p. cm.
Previously published: Nutrition for the healthy heart.
South Yarra, Victoria, Australia : Hardie Grant Books. 2001.
Includes bibliographical references and index.
ISBN 1-56924-557-6 (tradepaper)
1. Heart—Diseases—Nutritional aspects. 2. Heart—
Diseases—Diet therapy. 3. Nutrition. I. Title.

RC684.D5 S294 2002
616.1'20654—dc21   2002071866

9 8 7 6 5 4 3 2 1

Designed by Pauline Neuwirth, Neuwirth & Associates, Inc.
Printed in the Canada
Distributed by Publishers Group West

Contents

1

You and Your Heart

2

Eating for a Healthy Heart

Contents

3
Putting food to work for you

4
When diet isn't enough

5
Live your lifestyle

6
Recipes for the Healthy Heart

Contents

Author's thanks

Many people helped to bring this book together, and I am very grateful to them for their time and assistance.

First, I'm indebted to the health professionals who helped ensure that the information the book offers is up to date and reflects the latest research:

Lisa Yates, accredited practicing dietitian with a busy private practice in Sydney, Australia, edited the early versions of the manuscript, stressing the things that her clients always ask her and need to know.

Associate Professor Leon Simons, head of the lipid department, St. Vincent's Hospital, Darlinghurst, in New South Wales, Australia, helped with clinical background on heart disease and gave me good advice on the risk assessment quiz.

Susan Anderson, Food Information Program Manager, and Vanessa Jones, Public Health Nutritionist, both with the Australian Heart Foundation in New South Wales, provided wise counsel on the latest diet guidelines for fats and also helped with the food selection guide.

Dr. David Sullivan, from the Department of Clinical Biochemistry at Royal Prince Alfred Hospital, Camperdown, New South Wales, reviewed the section on medications and supplements and briefed me about the latest medical opinion on the management of blood lipids and dietary strategies.

Professor Andy Sinclair, head of food science at Royal Melbourne Institute of Technology in Australia, commented on the fats section at the eleventh hour.

Karen Kingham, accredited practicing dietitian and consultant, proofread the manuscript (more than once!), analyzed the recipes, and helped keep me going when things came unglued.

Author's Thanks

Carolyn Hankins, accredited practicing dietitian and consultant, also helped with recipe analyses and recipe testing.

Jennene Plummer, food consultant and editor of *Super Food Ideas* magazine, contributed recipes and cast her expert eye over the final batch.

Dr. Ron Bowery, Manager of R & D at Goodman Fielder Ltd in Australia, was—as always—a source of knowledge on fats and oils and current commercial manufacturing practices.

Second, thank you to two creative wordsmiths, who are the silent strength behind all good books:

Philippa Sandall, editorial consultant, colleague, and friend, helped direct the flow of the manuscript and steer me in the right direction when writer's block set in.

Clare Coney, editor, worked diligently to check and double-check all my writing and was a tower of strength when my energies were sapping. Nothing slips by her professional eye!

Third, thank you to all those people who spent time talking to me about their own heart problems and what sort of diet information they found helpful—John Penn, John Creagh, Nick Plummer, Jill Hooker, Mike Lillicrap, and Phillip Hurley.

Finally, to the team at Hardie Grant Books, including Sandie Grant, Julie Pinkham, and Tracy O'Shaughnessy, a big thank you for embracing me into their family of authors and accepting the metamorphosis of this book. They coped well when it started out small and ended up big!

Introduction

"Every calamity is a spur and valuable hint."
—Ralph Waldo Emerson, "Fate"

There's nothing like a personal problem to bring things into perspective! In other words, it's not until something happens to YOU that you truly realize the hurdles to face when you have to change the way you live—and eat! That's the reason why I began to write this book.

In my area of nutrition, I spend a lot of time writing about diet and healthy eating, I give talks on how to eat better, I go on the radio and answer people's questions about what's good and what's not, I analyze recipes for fat and fiber, and I occasionally work with food companies to create new products that are lighter and healthier. But this was always from a theoretical viewpoint—how to improve the eating habits of the "average" person.

One day, all that theory was put to the harsh test of reality. My husband, Dave, came home from the doctor with the news that he had high cholesterol. A routine checkup and blood test gave him a cholesterol reading of 242—not frighteningly high, but enough of a wake-up call.

We were both surprised. He was not overweight, but his hectic job involved long hours and traveling, which left little time for exercise. His diet was OK (being married to me!), but things had crept in along with a busy lifestyle—business dinners, drinks after work, the occasional bag of chips, pizza on Friday night after our son's basketball game. Still, we figured these extras should not have been a problem.

However, the doctor issued a warning. Dave was over 45, had a high-stress job, and his father had developed high cholesterol later in life. We sat down and worked through what he could change. It was a standard list any dietitian would give you, such as eating less saturated fat, less cholesterol, more fiber, more vegetables and fruit, less fast food and eating on the run.

I happened to mention some new research I'd been reading and how a handful of nuts a day could be beneficial for the heart. Dave was surprised. But aren't nuts high in fat? Aren't they fattening? Aren't they a no-no for anyone on a diet? What was it about nuts that made them good? Did they have to be eaten raw or roasted? I had to go back to the research and read up.

It was a turning point for him—and for me. He realized that there were some new things he could add to his meal plan rather than just eliminating "anything with fat." I realized how much research was buried in scientific journals, nutrition conferences, and dietitians' manuals. Not enough was getting out to the public, to doctors' rooms and magazines and newspapers.

It's not just the research on nuts that's new. Over the past five years, there's been lots of good news on soy, tea (along the lines of wine and antioxidants), vegetables and fruit, folate, whole grains, and low glycemic index carbohydrates—all foods that fall into the "eat more" category for a healthy heart diet.

Since then, I've interviewed dozens of others with high cholesterol levels or heart problems (these days it seems there are heaps of people over 40 facing these situations). They've told me what they would like to know in terms of food guides, menus, shopping tips, what to buy, what to choose when eating out, and how to figure out what's in food. All of this good, basic information I've incorporated into this book.

Dave found that making small changes to his usual way of eating, rather than drastically changing his whole diet, worked for him. He could get his cholesterol to drop by cutting out the mayo from his lunchtime sandwich, ordering fish more often when eating out, having a glass of wine but saying no to dessert, substituting nuts for chips with drinks, ordering more salads, switching to whole wheat bread, switching to low-fat milk. Little things, but they added up without a great deal of sacrifice.

If you are about to embark on a heart-healthy way of eating, be warned that it's not always easy. There's much conflicting advice from books, TV, alternative therapists, and well-meaning relatives who simply get it wrong. Not to mention the fact that genuine new research regularly surfaces to change the way professionals think about diet therapy. Some issues where the evidence is not clear cut—like the Mediterranean Diet or the desired ratio of protein to carbohydrate—can even divide the nutrition profession.

This book started out as a small pocket book of less than 80 pages. It's ended up as a standard-size book of over 200 pages, with a comprehensive guide to diet choices, meal ideas, food label advice, shopping lists, eating out tips, and recipes. To my way of thinking, that's a real testimony to the fact that changing food habits isn't as easy as we nutritionists often believe!

You'll find a general introduction to the causes of heart disease in Part One, along with a quick quiz that will give you insight into your own risk of heart problems. If you've already heard it or just want the food information, skip Part One and go straight to Part Two, which outlines the 10 steps for eating well.

Armed with the theory, you can then move on to Part Three, which takes you through the necessary ways to rethink your daily diet. You can take the menus and use them as templates, substituting similar foods that you prefer. You can mix and match the breakfast, lunch, and dinner suggestions, or adapt them to your own preferences. However, it's best if you eventually understand the hows and whys of nutrition and plan your own meals.

In Part Four, your options for medications are covered. In addition, the growing number of supplements is examined and their usefulness evaluated. To give you a balanced approach, Part Five gives advice on exercise (always important to good health), strategies to quit smoking, and ways to handle stress.

Part Six gives you 55 healthy recipes to get you started!

A final reminder: There are no shortcuts, no magic bullets, no single food or supplement that can lower cholesterol effortlessly or make your arteries clean and flexible again (although many promise to do so). It is the sum total of what you eat, combined with exercise, stress management, and a healthy lifestyle, that will make the difference.

I'm not "selling" you a diet like so many books do. Along with Dave's and my own experience, I've pulled together summaries of the scientific literature, hours of talking to academic and clinical specialists, tips from dietitians who deal with clients on the front lines, new recipes for the kitchen—all to come up with strategies that give you the best chance at lowering your cholesterol and looking after your heart in the years to come. I've tried to make it practical, easy-to-read, and helpful. I hope it is all that for you.

Good health,
Catherine Saxelby

For good general information on nutrition and healthy eating, visit Catherine's Web site at www.foodwatch.com.au.

What does it mean?
Your healthy heart at a glance

Medical terms can be confusing. Here's a quick guide to the most common medical jargon and what it means in plain English.

What your doctor says:	What your doctor really means:
Hyperlipidaemia	High levels of lipids or fats in the bloodstream, generally cholesterol or triglycerides
Hypercholesterolaemia	High levels of cholesterol (a type of fat) in the bloodstream
Arteriosclerosis	A general term meaning hardening of the arteries
Atherosclerosis	Thickening or "clogging" of the arteries due to an accumulation of tissue and fats, particularly cholesterol
HDL cholesterol	High-density lipoprotein cholesterol. Also known as the "good" cholesterol
Hypertension	High blood pressure (not stress or tension)
Hypertriglyceridaemia	High levels of triglycerides (a type of fat) in the bloodstream
LDL cholesterol	Low-density lipoprotein cholesterol. Also known as the "bad" cholesterol
Lipoprotein	Packets of fat with a coating or envelope of protein that carry lipids in the bloodstream
Myocardial infarction	Heart attack

What Does It Mean?

Obesity

Being very overweight, which puts you at risk of heart disease later in life

Platelet aggregation

Clumping together of tiny blood cells into a sticky mass that sticks to damaged blood vessels and collagen

Risk factor

Something that increases your chances of getting heart disease, like smoking or high cholesterol

Thrombosis

A clot in the blood which can partially or completely block an artery

PART 1

You and

Your Heart

TAKING STOCK—
A QUICK REFERENCE

Do you have high cholesterol? Have you just had a blood test and your doctor's told you you're a candidate for heart trouble? Do you come from a family with a history of heart complaints? Have you had a coronary bypass or heart attack?

If you answered yes to any of these questions, you know you're going to have to change the way you're eating and perhaps lose some weight.

Most of the illness and loss of life from heart disease can be prevented. Regular checks by your doctor, combined with a healthy diet and exercise, can do much to keep heart disease at bay.

Over the past 20 years, doctors have tested innovative drugs and discovered sophisticated new surgical techniques to bypass damaged arteries and remove blockages, but these are expensive treatments. The best way to prevent heart disease remains a healthy diet and physical activity (as well as quitting smoking).

HEART HEALTH FACTS

Heart disease is a major health problem. Even though death rates from heart disease have fallen in the past decade, it remains the leading cause of mortality in the U.S.

- Cardiovascular disease causes more deaths in both men and women than the next six leading causes of death combined.

- About 62 million Americans live with cardiovascular disease.
- There are almost 950,000 deaths annually from heart disease in the U.S.
- The disease includes high blood pressure, coronary heart disease (including heart attack and angina), stroke, congenital cardiovascular defects, and congestive heart failure, among others.
- The price tag: nearly $300 billion, including health spending (physicians, hospitals, medication, home health) and indirect costs such as lost productivity due to disability and death.
- Cardiovascular disease claims 58,000 more women than men each year.
- Among blacks, the risk of death from both stroke and high blood pressure is significantly higher than for whites.
- Striking differences in disease rates by both ethnicity and socioeconomic class underscore the need to improve screening and early detection for black and Mexican-American women, as well as women of lower socioeconomic status in all ethnic groups.
- Sudden cardiac deaths are increasing among young people (ages 15 to 34, with a 10 percent rise in the past decade. The increase is even higher among women and blacks.
- Despite health programs, many people are still at risk of heart disease because of smoking, blood pressure that's too high, eating the wrong foods, and being inactive. More and more of us are gaining weight while sport is rapidly becoming something we watch elite athletes do rather than participate in.

The good news is that much of the illness and death from heart disease is preventable. The key risk factors—smoking, high blood pressure, high cholesterol, overweight, and sedentary lifestyle—are all things you can improve or eliminate from your life.

What heart disease is that? An illness in many guises

Heart disease comes in many forms: myocardial infarction (heart attack), angina pectoris, hypertension (high blood pressure), heart failure, stroke, atherosclerosis (clogging of the arteries), thrombosis (blood clotting), and arrhythmia (irregular heartbeat).

But whatever form of heart disease you have—or are at risk of having—this book is for you, because for all forms of heart disease there are many things you can do to help yourself live a longer, healthier life and reduce your risk.

HOW THIS BOOK CAN HELP

This book will show you how to achieve a Healthy Heart diet, one that is low in fat, especially saturated fat, and rich in vegetables, fruit, and whole grains, along with plenty of protective antioxidants, vitamins, and minerals.

Coupled with regular exercise (like walking or swimming), this food plan will ensure you keep your heart in top condition and reverse any artery clogging that may have begun. Eating right and a healthy lifestyle will help save thousands of lives—especially lives lost prematurely by people in their 40s, 50s, and 60s with a lot more living to do! And it's not just about saving lives, but making sure your life is healthy and that you can enjoy it!

This book will show you how to make changes for the better to your meals and your daily routine. In addition, you will learn how to add "heart protector" foods to your daily diet and how to take advantage of functional foods like plant stanol esters, supplements, and alternative remedies.

If you have high cholesterol or raised blood pressure, you will find positive steps to take to reverse your condition. If you just want to avoid future trouble, there's lots of handy strategies to ward off heart disease in the years ahead.

Count the added benefits

Eating the healthy heart way:

- Makes losing weight easier (never easy but more achievable, particularly if you think long term, not just another quick-fix diet).
- Adds all-important vitamins, minerals, and antioxidants to your meals.
- Helps build strong bones.
- Helps keep blood pressure where it should be (without medications).
- Is suitable for those with diabetes, who are more likely to succumb to heart troubles.
- May keep cancer at bay, due to its bonus of antioxidants, fish, and low-fat meats.

Don't become a statistic! Start making changes to your food now. Your heart will thank you for it!

WHAT YOU NEED TO KNOW ABOUT RISK FACTORS

The causes of heart disease are many and varied. The American Heart Association and the American College of Cardiology have identified six major risk factors for heart trouble—some due to what we eat, some due to the way we live, some that we inherit from our parents and grandparents. If you have one of these factors, your chances of heart disease rise. For example, smoking or high blood pressure approximately doubles your coronary risk; having diabetes doubles the risk for men but raises it fourfold in women. As we grow older, our risk also rises. If you have two or more of these risk factors, your chances of developing a heart condition soar:

Proven Risk Factors

- Cigarette smoking
- High blood pressure
- High levels of total blood cholesterol and "bad" LDL cholesterol
- Low levels of "good" HDL cholesterol
- Diabetes
- Advancing years (over 50)

Suspected Risk Factors

There are six more risk factors for heart disease where the evidence is less strong, but they can significantly increase your personal risk depending on your circumstances. Some are called "indirect," as they affect one of the six proven factors. For example, if you're too heavy, this can raise blood pressure and cholesterol, which in turn raises the likelihood of a coronary event.

- Overweight, with most of your excess fat around your middle (abdominal fat or potbelly)
- Inactive (sedentary)
- Family history of early heart disease (before 60)
- Gender—risk is higher for males than females
- High blood levels of triglycerides
- High blood levels of homocysteine (see page 18)

For a quick assessment of your personal risk, try the checkup that follows.

GIVE YOURSELF A CHECKUP

Are you at risk of heart disease?

If you're worried about heart disease, see your doctor. To prepare yourself, work through this easy checkup, and see what your chances are. The questions relate to risk factors, conditions that increase the likelihood of heart disease. Assess yourself. Simply answer yes or no, and add up the number of yes answers at the end.

Part A: Proven risk factors

1. **Smoking**
   Do you smoke cigarettes, cigars, or a pipe?
   (a) Yes
   (b) No
2. **Blood pressure**
   Do you have high blood pressure?
   (a) Yes
   (b) No
3. **Blood cholesterol**
   Do you have high blood cholesterol? (Generally defined as 240 mg/dL or higher)
   (a) Yes
   (b) No
4. **HDL cholesterol**
   Do you have low HDL cholesterol? (Generally defined as less than 40 mg/dL for men and less than 50 mg/dL for women)
   (a) Yes
   (b) No
5. **Diabetes**
   Do you have diabetes (regardless of whether you are on pills, injections, or just manage by diet and exercise)?
   (a) Yes
   (b) No

6. **Age**
   Are you 50 years of age or older?
   (a) Yes
   (b) No

Part B: Suspected risk factors

7. **Weight**
   Do you consider yourself overweight?
   (a) Yes
   (b) No

8. **Body shape**
   If you're overweight, is most of your excess around your stomach/abdomen/midriff?
   (a) Yes
   (b) No

9. **Activity level**
   Are you inactive or do you have a sedentary job?
   (a) Yes
   (b) No

10. **Family history**
    Have any of your close relatives had heart problems (angina, high cholesterol) or died from heart disease (heart attack, stroke) before the age of 60?
    (a) Yes
    (b) No

11. **Gender**
    Are you male?
    (a) Yes
    (b) No

12. **Triglycerides**
    Do you have high blood triglycerides? (Generally defined as 200 mg/dL or higher)
    (a) Yes
    (b) No

There's More to Heart Health than Cholesterol

Your heart score

How did you score?

If you answered yes to any question in Part A:

You have a proven risk factor for heart disease. Don't delay. Make an appointment with your doctor to have a full checkup and start changing your diet and lifestyle today. This is particularly important if you answered yes to one or more questions in Part B; overweight, inactivity, and family history compound your risk. Even if you answered no to all Part B questions, you still have a proven risk factor that will need assessing.

If you answered no to all questions in Part A:

Your risk of heart troubles is not as great. But if you had one or more yes answers in Part B, you have risk factors that could become more critical as you grow older. Therefore, it's important to make prevention of heart disease a priority in your life. Read on to find out how to improve your diet and lifestyle now. In the years to come, your heart will thank you.

Regardless of your results, once you're over 50, make sure you get yourself assessed every few years by your doctor to stave off trouble.

If you answered no to all questions in Parts A and B:

It's unlikely that you're a candidate for future heart troubles. This quick quiz shows your chances of heart problems as low. Keep up the good work!

For an explanation of these key markers of heart health, read on.

CIGARETTE SMOKING

Smoking is deadly for the heart, being the sole cause of about 25 percent of the deaths due to heart disease. It triples the risk of dying from heart disease among middle-aged men and women. One in every five deaths in the U.S. is smoking related. Cigarette smoke contains at least 63 distinct cancer-causing chemicals, with the best understood being nicotine and carbon monoxide. According to the American Lung Association:

> ❧ Carbon monoxide binds with red blood cells, reducing the oxygen-carrying capacity of the blood. It literally robs your muscles, brain, and tissues of oxygen, making your whole body—especially your heart—work harder.
> ❧ Nicotine constricts blood vessels and reduces blood flow. Over time, it makes your airways narrow and allows less air into your lungs.

Together, the mixture of nicotine and carbon monoxide in each cigarette temporarily increases your heart rate and blood pressure, straining your heart and blood vessels.

Smoking also causes fatty deposits to form in blood vessels, which narrow and block them further, setting the scene for heart disease and stroke.

Since the 1990s, anti-tobacco advertisements have done much to bring down rates of smoking. But there are still an estimated 48 million cigarette smokers in the U.S., 4.5 million of whom are teenagers. And as smoking has declined among the white non-Hispanic population, tobacco companies have targeted African-Americans and Hispanics with intensive advertising campaigns.

HIGH BLOOD PRESSURE

What is blood pressure?

Blood pressure is a measure of the heart's force when pumping blood through the arteries. It is highest when the heart contracts (called the systolic measurement, around 120 mm/Hg in a healthy adult) and lowest when the heart relaxes (called the diastolic, at 80 mm/Hg). This is expressed as a normal blood pressure of 120/80.*

When it's high

High blood pressure (medically called hypertension) is a dangerous condition that raises your chance of suffering a stroke, heart attack, or kidney damage.

High blood pressure usually goes undetected until a medical checkup or—worst of all—when it unexpectedly causes a stroke or heart attack.

Once it was believed that our blood pressure rose automatically as we grew older and that this was a normal part of aging. Today, researchers believe that it need not happen if we lead a healthy lifestyle.

Your genes plus your lifestyle

There's no denying that the tendency to develop high blood pressure is something you inherit. If your parents had high blood pressure, then you are a likely candidate. But it's believed that the tendency will not appear unless one or more of the following five lifestyle factors trigger the mechanisms that cause high blood pressure.

---

*The first number, 120, refers to the systolic blood pressure, while the second number, 80, refers to the diastolic pressure.

1. Excess weight—forces the heart to pump harder
2. Heavy alcohol intake—responsible for about one in 10 blood pressure cases
3. High salt intake
4. Stress—but this can be lessened by relaxation techniques
5. Sedentary lifestyle

By following the 10-Step Plan in this book, you will cut back your calorie intake, which will help shed weight. More exercise will help you control your weight, aid in stress management, and give you a more active lifestyle. Along with cutting back on alcohol, these will assist in bringing down your high blood pressure.

What's high?

While things like your age and family history will influence your blood pressure, here's how the National Heart, Lung, and Blood Institute classifies blood pressure readings:

	SYSTOLIC	DIASTOLIC
Normal	130 or less	85 or less
High-normal	131–139	84–89
High	140 or more	90 or more

CHOLESTEROL

What is it?

Cholesterol is a white, waxy substance, a type of fat that is produced in the liver and released into the bloodstream. It is just one of a family of related substances known as sterols. Cholesterol is not bad—in the right amounts. A certain amount of it is needed by the body and has many uses.

> It acts as a building block for all cell membranes.
> It is required to produce sex hormones.
> It is required to make vitamin D.
> It forms the basis of bile acids, which help us digest fats.
> It is a part of the protective insulation around nerve fibers.

In other words, cholesterol is a normal and essential component of our bodies and the bodies of other animals.

Cholesterol transporters

Cholesterol is transported in the blood by a number of carrier molecules known as lipoproteins (lipid + protein). There are two main ones.

"Good" cholesterol

HDL cholesterol (HDL stands for high-density lipoprotein) is often referred to as the "good" cholesterol, as it ferries unwanted cholesterol back to the liver, where it is recycled or removed from the system as bile acids.

"Bad" cholesterol

LDL cholesterol (LDL stands for low-density lipoprotein) takes cholesterol from the liver. It is thought of as the "bad" cholesterol because, if it builds up, it can be deposited as fatty deposits on artery walls.

What is high cholesterol?

It depends to a degree on your own personal situation: whether you have heart disease, whether you fall into a high-risk group, or whether you're fairly healthy. The bottom line is to have your blood readings done and to talk to your doctor about your personal risk. Your doctor will guide you from there.

What to aim for

TOTAL CHOLESTEROL
> DESIRABLE: less than 200 mg/dL
> BORDERLINE: 200–239 mg/dL
> HIGH: 240 mg/dL or higher

LDL
> OPTIMAL: less than 100 mg/dL
> NEAR OPTIMAL: 100–129 mg/dL
> Borderline High: 130–159 mg/dL
> HIGH: 160–189 mg/dL
> VERY HIGH: 190 mg/dL or higher

HDL
> DESIRABLE, MEN: 40–50 mg/dL
> DESIRABLE, WOMEN: 50–60 mg/dL

Know your cholesterol ratio

There is a growing school of thought that says the ratio of total cholesterol to HDL is more accurate than total cholesterol alone as a marker for heart disease. Divide your total cholesterol reading by your HDL reading; ideally your calculation should equal 4 or less.

Did you know?

Cholesterol was named from two Greek words, *chole* (meaning bile) and *stereos* (meaning solid), because gallstones which are made from bile are composed of virtually pure cholesterol.

DIABETES AND INSULIN RESISTANCE
(THE METABOLIC SYNDROME)

Having diabetes increases the risk of heart disease two- to fourfold.

Diabetes is an illness in epidemic proportions in the U.S. and other Western countries. An estimated 16 million Americans have diabetes, at least one-third of whom are undiagnosed and untreated. And 20 to 30 million more have impaired glucose tolerance, or borderline diabetes.

Because many of the complications of diabetes—such as overweight, high triglycerides, high blood pressure, clotting and circulation problems—overlap with heart disease, researchers have coined the term the "Metabolic Syndrome" (formerly known as Syndrome X) to cover this cluster of problems.

Central to the Metabolic Syndrome is insulin resistance. The muscles become insensitive to insulin—the body produces insulin, but the tissues and muscles don't "recognize" it. The body then responds by making more insulin and so levels build up in the bloodstream. Sugars in the blood are unable to move into the muscles to generate energy, as insulin is needed to "unlock" the muscles to let it in.

The two problems—resistance to insulin and a high level of circulating fats in the blood—are related. No one knows for sure which comes first but, either way, a good diet and exercise will help both heart and diabetes ailments.

Losing excess weight around the stomach combined with regular exercise can lessen insulin resistance and improve the uptake of glucose by the muscles, which will prevent or slow the onset of diabetes.

Type 2 diabetes . . .

- Represents 85–90 percent of all cases of diabetes.
- The body fails to produce enough insulin or use the insulin it does produce to absorb sugars from food.
- Left untreated, the resulting high blood sugar levels can damage tiny blood vessels, thus reducing blood flow to the extremities, and can cause serious damage to the kidneys, nerves, skin, and eyes as well as increasing the risk of heart disease.
- It develops gradually, usually in adults over 40.
- It is influenced by unhealthy eating and lack of exercise.
- It is a progressive disease. Once you have it, you can only postpone, not prevent, its development. Diet and exercise, if not successful as treatment, can escalate into pills and eventually injections of insulin.

TRIGLYCERIDES

What are triglycerides?

Triglycerides is really a technical word for all fats and includes the fat that circulates in the bloodstream, the fat from the food we eat, and the fat produced by the body, mainly in the liver.

On their own, high triglycerides aren't as strong a risk factor for heart disease as high cholesterol. But your doctor will take more notice of them if you already have heart disease or have other risk factors like a family history of heart problems, high blood pressure, are a smoker, have diabetes, or are overweight.

Quite commonly, a high triglyceride reading is related to having diabetes or to being overweight, drinking too much alcohol, or to certain inherited metabolic conditions.

What's high?

The standard recommended goal for triglycerides is 200 mg/DL or lower, though evidence is suggesting this may be too high and that levels over 100 mg/dL may predict an increased risk of heart disease.

If you discover that your triglyceride level is too high, the 10-Step Plan outlined in this book—losing weight, cutting back on saturated fats, doing more exercise—will help.

But in addition, there are two key factors that you may want to consider if high triglycerides are your main heart problem:

❯ Eat more omega-3 fatty acids from fish (see Step 6), or perhaps talk to your doctor about fish oil capsules (see page 108).

❯ Limit alcohol.

Your doctor or dietitian can advise you.

HOMOCYSTEINE

A high level of homocysteine in the blood is now being recognized as a new, independent risk factor for heart troubles.

If the level of homocysteine in your blood is too high, the chances of blood vessel damage and atherosclerosis are also high, in much the same way that high blood levels of cholesterol can predict how likely you are to have heart disease.

For years, doctors puzzled as to why some people succumb to heart attack when they have no known risk factors—they don't smoke, their blood fats are within safe limits, they have no family history of heart problems or high blood pressure, they are not overweight.

Now, with the discovery of homocysteine, an explanation is here. One of the clues was that people with a rare inherited disease known as homocysteinaemia (deficiency of the enzyme cystathionine synthase), which led to raised levels of homocysteine, often died early in life from heart disease.

But the good news is that a high level of homocysteine can be treated with modifications to your daily diet or by supplementation.

What is it?

Homocysteine is an amino acid produced by the body. It is part of a biochemical cycle and is converted to methionine.

For this cycle to function, folate and its close relatives vitamins B_{12} and B_6 are needed to activate the pathway. If you are getting plenty of folate, B_6, and B_{12} from your food, they "detoxify" the homocysteine, driving levels down and keeping you safe from heart troubles.

But if there is not enough folate, B_{12}, and B_6 in your diet, the homocysteine builds up in the blood and can start a slow accumulation of plaque on artery walls. There's also evidence that it makes the blood more likely to clot.

2
PART

Eating for a

Healthy Heart

Eating for a healthy heart will not only be doing your heart good, but these same ideas can help you lose weight, improve your overall health, and make diabetes (if you have it) easier to manage. It's a way of eating you can follow for the rest of your life.

THE 10-STEP PLAN TO EATING FOR A HEALTHY HEART

The 10 steps that I describe are based on the latest nutrition research and recommendations from health authorities like the Centers for Disease Control and Prevention (CDC) and the American Heart Association. While there's some debate about the relative priority of each principle (for example, some researchers feel salt is less of an issue than a good supply of antioxidants), nutritionists agree that they're all good guiding rules.

The steps are based on three principles:

- Shedding fat (Step 1)
- Focusing on the fats in your diet (Steps 2–6)
- Harnessing the power of plants (Steps 7–10)

Here are the 10 steps:
1. Shed excess body fat, especially if it's around your stomach.
2. Cut back on saturated fats and trans fats.
3. Make sure the fats you do eat are unsaturated.
4. Add plant stanol esters to your diet.
5. Cut back on cholesterol from food.

6. Boost your omega-3s.
7. Sweep cholesterol away with soluble fiber.
8. Eat more folate.
9. Up the antioxidants.
10. Add the heart protectors—soy, nuts, and whole grains.

S T E P

1

SHED EXCESS BODY FAT, ESPECIALLY IF IT'S AROUND YOUR STOMACH

This is the first and most important step. If you are carrying more weight (body fat) than you should, your heart has to pump harder. Obesity tends to raise your blood cholesterol, triglycerides, and blood pressure too.

If most of your excess is around your middle—which scientists call abdominal fat—you're more likely to develop heart disease and diabetes. It seems the fat stored around the stomach or abdomen is more "active" and enters the bloodstream more readily than fat from hips and thighs.

Having more rounded hips and thighs (the pear shape of many women) is not a hazard for your heart, which is one of the reasons why men—who tend to carry fat as a beer gut or potbelly—are more likely to suffer heart attacks than women. But if your waist is larger than your hips, you're at increased risk of heart disease.

For many people, simply shedding that spare tire will bring down cholesterol and normalize blood pressure—even if the loss is just 10 or so pounds, rather than down to your ideal body weight. One of the best ways to avoid heart problems later in life is to maintain your weight so you don't put on fat around the middle.

You should approach this in two ways. First, aim to cut back your total calorie intake by cutting back on saturated fats and alcohol. If you follow the plan outlined here, your diet will automatically be shaped this way. Second, aim to burn more calories by doing more exercise and building up metabolically active muscle via weight training. You'll be helping your heart and your weight at the same time.

Finally, it must be recognized that some thin people eat all the right foods yet still battle to keep their cholesterol low. If this is you, your doctor will guide you and may suggest a trial of cholesterol-lowering medications (see page 105).

S T E P

2

CUT BACK ON SATURATED FATS AND TRANS FATS

Focus on fats

Fats play a big role in heart health. If you can get your fat intake right, it will make a huge difference. Cut back on saturated and trans fats, while making any fats you do eat the unsaturated kind, i.e. monounsaturated and polyunsaturated. Remember that if you need to lose weight, the easiest way to cut back on calories is to drop your overall fat (and alcohol) intake.

Cutting back on saturated and trans fats will help lessen the fatty buildup on blood vessel walls and lower your cholesterol (both total cholesterol and bad LDL cholesterol). It's also a key to losing body fat.

Aim for:

➤ less saturated fat, no more than 14 g a day for the average moderately active person.

Saturated fats

These are found in:

➤ Animal foods such as butter, cream, fatty cuts of meat, poultry skin, whole cheese, whole and 2% milk, and premium ice cream.

➤ Deep-fried fast food (fries, fried chicken), salty snack foods, and pastries and cookies that are made using palm oil, a saturated oil or hydrogenated commercial fats.

What they do:

Saturated fats tend to raise both total cholesterol and LDL. We need to keep this type of fat to a minimum in our diet.

Trans fats

Trans fats or trans fatty acids (TFAs), are a minor type of fat. They are found in:

➤ Processed foods (cookies, crackers, snack cakes, frozen entrées)

➤ Fried fast foods

➤ Some hard margarines and commercial solidified fats made for baking and pastry. The trans fats are formed during hydrogenation (hardening) of vegetable oils to turn them into a more solid spread. Any fat-free margerine or spread is usually a good alternative.

What they do:

Raise LDL cholesterol in the same way as saturated fats. We need to limit this type of fat.

How your fat intake should be divided

No more than 30 percent of total calories from fat

▶ 7 to 10 percent from saturated fats
▶ 10 to 15 percent from monounsaturated fats
▶ 10 percent from polyunsaturated fats
▶ Cut out all trans fats if possible

S T E P

3

MAKE SURE THE FATS YOU EAT ARE UNSATURATED

Unsaturated fats include both the mono- and polyunsaturated fats found in oils, spreads, most nuts, seeds, and avocado. Both types are preferred over saturated fats, and both lower cholesterol, thus cutting your risk of having a heart attack. If you follow the advice here, you'll automatically consume more unsaturated fats.

Aim for:

▶ Polyunsaturates—around 20 g a day in a 1,800-calorie diet.

> Monounsaturates—a minimum 30 g a day in a 1,800-calorie diet.

❥ HEART MYTHS

WHAT YOU'VE HEARD: Olive oil is the only oil to use if you're trying to stop heart disease.

FACT: Olive oil is a good choice, but another monounsaturated option is canola oil (which adds a bonus of omega-3 fatty acids). Extra-virgin cold-pressed olive oil contains a range of antioxidants that are helpful to include in the diet and that give it the edge over other oils. But it is more expensive and strong-flavored (see page 60).

WHAT YOU'VE HEARD: Vegetable oils keep your fat intake low.

FACT: Vegetable oils (corn, safflower, sunflower, soybean), though light in flavor and color, are not good heart-healthy choices.

WHAT YOU'VE HEARD: Avocados are full of fat and thus are bad for the heart.

FACT: Avocados ARE high in fat (at 23 percent, or 22 g from half a medium avocado). But their fat is rich in monounsaturates that, like olive and canola oil, are now regarded as a healthy fat for the heart. Like other fruits and vegetables, avocados contain no cholesterol.

THE GOOD FAT GUIDE

When it comes to cholesterol and the heart, not all fats are bad. Saturated and trans fats are the coronary culprits, as they tend to raise your blood cholesterol and clog and stiffen arteries, but mono- and polyunsaturated fats are beneficial. Read on for an update.

The good ones

Monounsaturated

Found in:
- Olive oil and canola oil
- Margarines made from olive and canola oils
- Avocados
- Nuts, particularly macadamias, pecans, pistachios, almonds, peanuts, and cashews

Monounsaturates reduce levels of harmful LDL cholesterol in the blood, but not to the same extent as the omega-6 polyunsaturates. However, there is some evidence that monounsaturates can lower insulin resistance and decrease heart disease. They also tend to be more stable and less likely to oxidize than polyunsaturates, so they draw less on your body's own antioxidants. They should make up the majority of fats in your diet.

Polyunsaturated

These occur in two forms, both of which your body needs for good health.

Omega-6 polyunsaturates

Found in:
- Oils like sunflower, safflower, soybean, cottonseed, maize, sesame, and grape seed
- Polyunsaturated margarines
- Wheat germ
- Lecithin
- Rice bran, oats
- Nuts, particularly Brazil nuts, walnuts, pine nuts, sesame seeds

Omega-6 polyunsaturated fats are very effective at reducing both total cholesterol and LDL and have been a cornerstone of diets— replacing saturated fats from butter—since the 1960s. Small quantities are important for the heart, but we don't need lots of them.

As a group, these fats usually occur in oils accompanied by vitamin E, which helps stabilize their structure and acts as their own antioxidant.

Omega-3 polyunsaturates

Found in:
- Fish, especially oily fish (herring, salmon, tuna, mackerel, sardines)
- Seafood
- Very lean red meat, venison
- Liver, kidneys
- A simpler version is found in flaxseed (linseed) oil, canola oil, walnuts, pecans, omega-enriched eggs, soybeans, green vegetables, herbs, and wild greens (like purslane)

Omega-3s reduce the tendency for the blood to clot and protect against arrhythmia; they lower triglycerides and may lower high blood pressure (see page 108).

S T E P

4

ADD PLANT STANOL ESTERS TO YOUR DIET

Plant stanol esters (phytosterols) are a group of natural compounds with a similar structure to cholesterol, yet they have the ability to inhibit its absorption from the digestive tract into the body.

To be absorbed, cholesterol normally mixes with other substances to form a tiny particle that is known as a micelle, which then allows it to pass into the bloodstream. Plant stanol esters, because they are closely related to cholesterol, actually compete with cholesterol for a place in the micelle. If a cholesterol molecule can't find a place in the micelle, it is not absorbed and simply passes out of the body with other bowel wastes. It has been proven that stanol esters, if eaten in sufficiently high quantities, lower blood cholesterol, particularly LDL.

Plant stanol esters in the food supply

Stanol esters are found in most plant foods. The greatest amounts occur in vegetable oils, with smaller amounts in nuts, legumes, breads, and cereal grains, and still smaller amounts in fruits and vegetables. In an average diet, we regularly take in between 0.2 and 0.6 g of stanol esters a day, but this level is too low to have any noticeable effect on our cholesterol.

Plant stanol esters, extracted and concentrated during the processing of soy or wood pulp, are now being added to spreads and salad dressings.

Effectiveness of plant stanol esters

There are good clinical trials showing that plant stanol esters are effective at reducing blood cholesterol levels. According to the FDA, three servings per day can mean a cholesterol reduction of as much as 20 points.

If you already use a spread, it makes good sense to swap it for one with plant stanol esters (for example, Benecol or Take Charge). While they cost more than other spreads, the good news is that they're low-sodium, made from good oils, and will complement any medications (such as a statin to lower cholesterol) that you may be taking. Also, if you normally drink a reduced-fat milk, it's worth swapping that for a special stanol ester variety. Look out for other similarly enhanced dairy foods.

Even if you ate no cholesterol at all (say if you were a vegan), you would still have it circulating in your blood. Our bodies produce cholesterol—known as endogenous cholesterol—for use in many bodily functions. Endogenous cholesterol enters the digestive tract via bile and would normally be reabsorbed and then transported to the liver, where it could be recycled. Once you start eating plant stanol esters, they reduce the absorption of all cholesterol in the digestive tract, which includes that from bile. This means that in addition to lowering the cholesterol you absorb from your diet, plant stanol esters have the potential to reduce your cholesterol further by limiting the absorption of your body's own cholesterol.

Remember, however, that plant stanol esters will work best when included with two or three of your daily meals, and they will only work as long as you keep eating them. Once you stop, your blood cholesterol will return to previous levels.

Safety aspects

Plant stanol esters have been shown to be safe even when consumed at high levels (say over 5 g a day) for long periods of time. They have been used in pharmaceuticals since the 1950s, when sterol esters were prescribed to control high cholesterol. No adverse side effects were reported at doses as high as 30 g a day—fifteen times that suggested today for heart health. There is no significant benefit in taking more than 2–3 g daily, but if you did this is not a health risk: Plant stanol esters are poorly absorbed by the body and are rapidly excreted.

The main safety concern has been for fat-soluble vitamins and antioxidants—beta-carotene and the related carotenoids—which were thought to be affected by stanol esters consumption. But clinical trials showed little effect on fat-soluble vitamins, and the observed decreases in carotenoids stayed within the normal range. However, as a precaution, the American Heart Association recommends that yellow and orange fruits and vegetables (high in beta-carotene) be included in your diet regularly if you eat foods containing plant stanol esters.

The only people who should not eat stanol esters are those with a rare inherited genetic disorder called homozygous sitosterolaemia, a condition in which plant stanol esters are absorbed quite readily from the intestine. This is the opposite of most people; plant stanol esters are generally not well absorbed. Homozygous sitosterolaemia can result in heart disease at a young age. However, it is extremely rare, occurring in only one in 6 million people.

Plant stanol esters should be viewed as an additional weapon in the war against cholesterol. They are not a substitute for your medication, nor are they a replacement for a healthy diet. But they will work in addition to both—it's a situation where the final effect is greater than the sum of the two parts.

Aim for:
- 2–3 servings of plant stanol ester-enriched foods each day (although lower intakes are still effective for some people).

Foods containing plant stanol esters	Stanol esters per serving (g)
2 teaspoons stanol ester spread (e.g. Benecol, Take Charge)	0.8
1 glass (8 oz) milk with stanol esters	0.8
1 container (8 oz) yogurt with stanol esters	0.8
1 serving mayonnaise or dressing with stanol esters	0.8

STEP

5

CUT BACK ON CHOLESTEROL

If you have high blood cholesterol or are at risk of heart disease, it's best to minimize the amount of cholesterol you eat.

When some people eat a lot of cholesterol, it pushes up the amounts of cholesterol circulating in their blood. In contrast, most healthy people simply adjust their internal production to produce less, or they eliminate more cholesterol when they eat more of it, so a steady blood level is maintained.

However, even if your general blood cholesterol level doesn't change, the temporary enrichment of blood fats with cholesterol after a meal can still cause damage, which is why doctors restrict cholesterol.

The good news is that if your diet has a little more high-cholesterol food than desired, this can be counteracted by adding plant stanol esters to your diet.

Cholesterol countdown

All animal foods (meat, fish, chicken, eggs, milk) have some cholesterol, while plant foods (vegetables, nuts, beans, pasta) contain none.

The richest sources of cholesterol are organ meats like kidney, eggs, and seafood like prawns and squid.

Cholesterol in foods

High (greater than 200 mg per serving)

Kidney
Prawns, squid (calamari)
Medium (100–200 mg per serving)
Eggs (includes eggs in dishes like puddings and meatloaf)
Crab, lobster
Modest (less than 100 mg per serving)
Liver
Oysters, scallops, mussels, octopus
Fish, canned tuna, canned salmon
Lean beef, lamb, pork, chicken

 # HEART MYTHS

HOW MANY EGGS CAN I EAT?

Eggs are probably the one food people miss most on cholesterol-lowering plans. But at around 200 mg/dL an egg, they are fairly high in cholesterol. (All the cholesterol is concentrated in the yolk; the white has virtually none.)

If you have high cholesterol or diabetes or are overweight, up to four eggs a week is permissible. Otherwise, up to seven a week is fine.

One egg has around 6 g of fat total, of which only 2 g is saturated fat, with 4 g being monounsaturated and 0.5 g being polyunsaturated. In comparison, a slice of Cheddar cheese has more than 10 g of fat, of which about 6 g is saturated.

Omega-3 enriched eggs have the same cholesterol and total fat as ordinary eggs, but due to the special feed given to the hens, the type of fat in the egg contains more omega-3 and less saturated fat. They are a better choice.

6

BOOST YOUR OMEGA-3S

Omega-3s are a must for a healthy heart. While they have no effect on cholesterol, they have many other benefits:

- Steady the heart's rhythm and minimize cardiac arrhythmia—chaotic and irregular heartbeats—which is often fatal
- Keep the blood free flowing, especially through small blood vessels
- Lower triglyceride levels in the blood
- Lower blood pressure
- Slow the buildup of fatty material on the inner walls of blood vessels
- Prevent platelets in the blood from clumping together, thus reducing the chances of blood clots (an action similar to aspirin)
- Make the arteries more elastic

Omega-3s are found in all fish and seafood but particularly in oily fish such as salmon, tuna, sardines, mackerel, and herring (both fresh and canned). However, to reach a clinical effect quickly, your doctor may recommend a course of fish oil capsules (see page 108).

Aim:
- to eat two or three fish meals a week
- to use oils or spreads that contain omega-3s

Ways with omega-3s

🍤 Pan-fry, barbecue, or bake fresh fish in place of meat for meals. Make a habit of going to a fish market or good fish shop regularly, and you'll be tempted to cook fish more often.

🍤 If you dislike cooking fish at home, make a point of ordering fish when you eat out. Seafood like oysters and steamed scallops are light and delicious.

🍤 Keep a supply of canned salmon, tuna, and sardines in the kitchen for quick sandwich fillings or salads.

🍤 Choose oils that add omega-3s to your cooking, like flaxseed and canola.

🍤 Look for omega-enriched eggs.

🍤 Eat plenty of vegetables, especially the dark-green types.

🍤 Include flaxseeds in muffins and homemade bread.

🍤 Include walnuts and pecans in baking, or sprinkle them on breakfast cereal and salads for more omega-3s.

🍤 HEART MYTHS

What you've heard: Buying foods labeled NO CHOLES-TEROL is the key to lowering your cholesterol.

Fact: Foods that advertise themselves as containing no cholesterol are only useful if they're also low in saturated fat. Unfortunately, many are not. Foods such as potato chips and crackers are free of cholesterol, but they contain a saturated fat like palm oil or hydrogenated soybean oil—which is not going to benefit your heart. Cholesterol is only found in animal products, so there's none in any vegetable oil (see page 72).

STEP

7

SWEEP CHOLESTEROL AWAY
WITH SOLUBLE FIBER

In contrast to what you can achieve by cutting back on saturated and trans fats, the effect of soluble fiber on blood cholesterol is mild. Nevertheless it is part of the cumulative approach of the 10-Step Plan.

Oat bran, along with barley, rice bran, and psyllium have at various times enjoyed publicity for their heart-saving properties. Their beta-glucan, a gummy type of soluble fiber, can bind bile acids (end products of cholesterol metabolism) and sweep them out of the body in the feces. This prevents them from re-entering the bloodstream and lowers the level of cholesterol circulating in the blood.

Scientists have calculated that by including 3 g of soluble fiber in your diet a day, you can decrease your cholesterol by 2 to 3 percent. This means eating three apples or three servings of oats. Don't forget that psyllium, wheat germ, barley, and legumes (soybeans, soy flour, lentils) are also good sources of soluble fiber. All vegetables and fruit have some, with pectin-rich types such as oranges, grapefruit, apples, and dried fruit (prunes, raisins) being the richest.

Aim for:
- 2–3 servings of foods containing soluble fiber a day.

Ways to eat more soluble fiber

- Choose a cereal made from oats, barley, or psyllium. Psyllium is the husk or outer coating of the plantago seed and contains eight times more soluble fiber than oat bran. Research proves it has a much stronger effect on cholesterol than oat bran. You can buy it as raw flakes of psyllium at health food shops (it looks like fine wheat bran), or look for cereal made from it.

- Sprinkle some oat bran, barley bran, rice bran, raw psyllium, or wheat germ over your usual cereal.
- Add raw psyllium flakes or oat bran to muffins and cakes in place of half the flour.
- Add a few tablespoons of oat bran or psyllium to a low-fat smoothie.
- Increase your intake of beans and lentils—baked beans on toast is a quick and nutritious light meal.
- Use canned beans in salads or tossed with pasta.
- Add beans or lentils to soups, curries, and stews.

Harness the power of plants

Only in recent years has the power of the plant kingdom come to be appreciated by nutritionists. Yes, everyone's mother and grandmother knew how good those vegetables and whole grains were for us, but it wasn't until research into antioxidants started to gear up that it became apparent that plants hold a unique place in our diet. The number of natural phytochemicals they contain, along with their vitamins, minerals, fiber, and essential fatty acids, puts them in a special category of their own. Vegetables, nuts, whole grains, seeds, beans, and fruit offer us so much. You can start to tap in to their power and put it to use to help your heart.

STEP

8

EAT MORE FOLATE

Folate, a B vitamin, has been in the news for its ability to prevent birth defects such as spina bifida, but what you may not realize is how vital it is to a Healthy Heart. Eating plenty of folate is an important way of keeping homocysteine levels in the blood down (see page 19). In fact, folate may turn out to be one of the underlying explanations for why a healthy diet with plenty of vegetables, fruit, and whole grains (all sources of folate) can lower rates of heart disease.

Aim for:
- ❥ Plenty of vegetables, fruits, folate-fortified cereals, whole grain breads and pasta.

Tips for eating more folate

- ❥ Aim to eat at least two pieces of fresh fruit a day. Fruits rich in folate are citrus (oranges, lemons, grapefruit) and berries (strawberries, blueberries, blackberries).
- ❥ Aim for at least five servings of vegetables and salad a day. Dark-green vegetables such as spinach and broccoli, and Asian greens such as bok choy are the best, but vegetables like asparagus, avocado, herbs, and dark salad leaves (watercress, for example) are also good.
- ❥ Folate is extremely sensitive to light, heat, and air. It is easily destroyed during cooking, so eating a fresh salad each day makes good sense.
- ❥ Use avocado as a spread or with salad or pasta.

- Look for a breakfast cereal that's been fortified with folate (check the ingredients list or nutrition panel—most highlight folate on the pack). Generally a bowl provides 50–100 micrograms. The Recommended Dietary Allowance (RDA) for adults and children over 18 is 400 micograms. Women who are pregnant or planning to become pregnant need 600 micrograms a day. (Note that 1 microgram of folate = 0.6 micrograms of folic acid from supplements and fortified foods.)
- Opt for whole grain cereal. Or sprinkle 1–2 tablespoons of wheat germ over other cereals.
- Switch to whole grain bread instead of white.
- Have a serving of lean meat.
- Eat a handful of unsalted nuts (particularly peanuts) as a snack.
- Drink tea rather than coffee—it's moderately high in folate.

STEP

9

UP THE ANTIOXIDANTS

Scientists are turning to antioxidants to see if they can protect against heart disease by preventing bad LDL cholesterol from being oxidized.

Oxidized LDL

If the level of LDL cholesterol in the body builds up over and above what is needed (and if you don't eat enough antioxidants), it is more likely to be oxidized—reacting with oxygen to form a slightly different substance. Once it's oxidized, LDL cholesterol starts to cause problems, as the oxidized form is easily deposited as a fatty plaque layer inside blood vessel walls, where it can narrow or block them.

The oxidized LDL plaque can also act as an irritant that summons white blood cells to fight off the "infection." This can eventually trigger a chain reaction, producing a real inflammation that may erupt suddenly and block an artery. Or over time the plaque may leave scar tissue, which gradually thickens and blocks blood flow through critical arteries.

How antioxidants work

Antioxidants are molecules which act as part of the body's defense network. They destroy substances called free radicals that occur naturally in our bodies; free radicals are also left behind by smog, cigarette smoke, the sun's radiation, and other chemicals.

Free radicals cause damage to cell membranes, DNA genetic material, and fatty acids through the process of oxidation, in much the same way that air turns a cut apple brown or rusts a nail.

If you don't consume enough antioxidants, researchers now believe that free radicals can dominate and initiate the damage to fats that is the beginning of heart disease.

For the heart, the best-known antioxidant is vitamin E. But it works best in a team of other protective antioxidants, such as vitamin C, ubiquinone (co-enzyme Q10), and selenium.

In addition, many naturally occurring antioxidants—termed phytochemicals—play a role. These you won't find in supplements. They include carotenoids, flavonoids, isoflavones, catechins, and lignans. Some of these—like the catechins in tea, red wine, and chocolate—are more powerful scavengers of free radicals than the well-studied beta-carotene and vitamin C.

In this book, you'll find many foods such as vegetables, fruit, wine, tea, and whole grains recommended for their high level of these powerful antioxidants. Don't ignore them!

Vegetables and fruits

More than 200 studies have shown that people who consume lots of vegetables and fruit have a lower risk of heart attack and stroke than those who don't. Originally, researchers believed this was due to the high content of antioxidant vitamins in fresh produce—like beta-carotene and vitamins C and E—but now they attribute it to other natural plant compounds, the phytochemicals, which appear to have an even more powerful antioxidant capacity.

Produce with the strongest potential for lowering heart problems are:

- Cruciferous vegetables like broccoli, brussels sprouts, cauliflower, cabbage, and turnips
- Leafy green vegetables like spinach and kale and dark lettuces and salad leaves
- Citrus fruit like oranges, lemons, grapefruit, and tangelos.

For an easy guide to these handy phytochemicals, see the table on pages 45–46.

Eating plenty of these foods is the key to heart health—and they also give you the bonus of folate, which keeps homocysteine low.

Aim for:
- 5 or more servings of vegetables a day
- 2 or more servings of fruit a day

Tips for increasing your intake of vegetables and fruits
- Snack on fruit instead of crackers or chips. Try to bring a couple of pieces to work so you eat them over the course of the day.

❥ Finish meals with sliced fruit or a fruit salad.

❥ Serve two or three different vegetables with dinner.

❥ Try to eat a tossed green salad every day. Make it with darker lettuce leaves, and add some fresh herbs like mint or watercress.

❥ Add greens to your sandwiches.

❥ Cook a vegetarian meal once or twice a week.

❥ In winter, cook up hearty vegetable soups such as minestrone, pumpkin, pea, cauliflower, or spinach.

❥ Serve vegetables char-grilled or barbecued. Good ones to use are zucchini, tomato halves, bell pepper, eggplant, parsnip, sweet potato, and onion.

❥ Serve vegetable sticks with low-fat dips instead of corn chips or crackers.

Eat by the rainbow

Choose a wide variety of brightly colored vegetables and fruit. Color is usually a sign of phytochemicals being present. For example, opt for pumpkin or sweet potato rather than the normal white potato, buy romaine lettuce instead of the pale iceberg, purple Spanish onion instead of white, dark red grapes instead of white, and red cabbage over green. This doesn't mean you never eat the paler types, but variety is the key.

The good antioxidant guide

Here is a sample list (by no means complete) of the main types of antioxidants and where they occur in food.

Antioxidant	Main food sources	Benefit
Beta-carotene	Carrots, pumpkin, apricots, mango and other yellow-orange produce	Orange, yellow pigment in plants; inhibits the early stages of tumor development; improves immune function
Lycopene	Tomato, ruby grapefruit, watermelon, mango	Red pigment in plants; may cut risk of prostate cancer
Lutein	Spinach	Protects the macula of the eye from degeneration, a common loss of vision in older adults
Vitamin C	Fruit, fruit juices, and vegetables. The best sources are citrus fruit, guava, kiwifruit, berries, (strawberries, raspberries, black currants, etc.), mango, bell peppers, parsley, broccoli, spinach, pineapple, and cabbage.	Inhibits cancer-causing nitrosamine formation; reduces cancers of the digestive tract; regenerates vitamin E
Vitamin E	Oils (sunflower, cottonseed, canola), nuts, wheat germ, margarines, and whole grains. Added to fish oil tablets to keep them stable.	Protects polyunsaturated fats and beta-carotene from being oxidized (broken down); helps maintain the stability of the fats in cell membranes
Catechins	Tea	May help protect against heart disease, skin cancer, and stomach cancer
Flavonoids	Tea, wine, grapes, apples, onions, berries, lemons, limes, oranges	Minimize the oxidation of LDL cholesterol
Anthocyanins	Berries (blueberries, cranberries, bilberries, black currants), black grapes, black cherries.	Blue, purple, and red pigments in plants; antioxidants; mild anti-bacterial effect— cranberries can prevent urinary tract infections

Indoles	Broccoli, cabbage, cauliflower, brussels sprouts, Chinese cabbage, mustard	Trigger the release of anti-cancer enzymes; can reduce tumor development
Allium sulphur compounds	Garlic, onion, leeks	Help neutralize carcinogens; anti-bacterial
Isoflavones	Soybeans, other beans, tofu, tempeh, soy milk, lentils, peas	May relieve hot flashes and other menopausal symptoms; may reduce risk of breast and prostate cancers; helps prevent osteoporosis
Lignans	Flaxseeds, sesame seeds, bran, whole grains, beans, vegetables	Similar to isoflavones
Selenium	Seafood, liver, kidney, lean meat, whole grains	Enhances immune response and affects DNA repair, which can prevent the development and growth of cancer; works in combination with vitamins C and E
Zinc	Seafood (especially oysters), lean meat, chicken, milk, whole grains, dried beans, lentils, and nuts	Part of the key enzyme superoxide dismutase, which neutralizes free radicals

10

ADD THE HEART PROTECTORS

Research is unearthing a whole host of foods that actually work to protect your heart. These include soy, nuts, and whole grains, as well as vegetables and fruits. All bring with them a wide range of natural plant antioxidants, "healthy" fats, vitamin E, folate, plus a number of often-unknown substances. Whatever the active agents turn out to be, all these foods are nutritious, delicious, and worth having in your meals.

Super soy

Soy is one explanation for the low rates of heart disease in Japanese and Chinese populations, where soy foods have been staples for centuries. A key study which analysed 38 well-run clinical trials on the effect of eating soy protein instead of animal protein was published in the *New England Journal of Medicine* in 1995. It found that for those who ate soy products like tofu or soy milk, cholesterol levels were reduced by around 9 percent, LDL cholesterol by nearly 13 percent, and triglycerides by about 10 percent. Interestingly, people with normal cholesterol levels showed no effects when adding soy to their diet, but those with moderate to high levels did benefit.

In a U.S. clinical trial reported in the *American Journal of Clinical Nutrition*, men who ate a low-fat diet and relied on soy as their main protein source for 5 weeks saw their LDL decrease by as much as 14 percent and their HDL increase by as much as 8 percent. Men who ate low-fat diets but relied on meat for protein also saw cholesterol improvements, but not nearly as much as the soy eaters.

How does soy work?

In addition to soy protein's ability to lower cholesterol, soy contains isoflavones such as daidzein and genistein that work as antioxidants to stop LDL cholesterol from being oxidized. They also keep blood vessels more elastic and able to flex with pressure, as well as preventing blood clots from forming.

And don't forget that soy contains a lot of soluble fiber which, like oat bran, removes excess cholesterol from your digestive system.

In November 1999, the FDA approved a health claim allowing soy foods in the U.S. to carry a label stating that, as part of a diet low in saturated fat and cholesterol, 25 g of soy protein a day could reduce the risk of heart disease. Foods must have at least 6.25 g of soy protein in a serving before a food can make a claim on the packaging.

Aim for:
- 25 g of soy protein a day (equivalent to 3–4 servings of soy foods)

How to add soy protein to your diet

- Swap low-fat milk for low-fat soy drinks on cereal or in smoothies.
- Add canned drained soybeans to curries and soups.
- Make nachos with soybeans in place of kidney beans.
- Drain firm tofu, and slice into strips or cubes; marinate and add to stir-fries or soups.
- Buy soy snacks.
- Substitute defatted soy flour for one-third of the ordinary wheat flour when baking muffins and cakes.
- Try a frozen vegetarian option based on soy slices, medallions, or burgers.
- Use soft tofu (which has the consistency of mayonnaise) to make sauces or a creamy salad dressing.

Go nuts

A handful of nuts a day now has the blessing of nutritionists, thanks to almost a dozen recent studies.

For example, in California, a Seventh Day Adventist health study tracked more than 30,000 people for 6 years and found that those who ate nuts more than four times a week had 50 percent fewer heart attacks (both fatal and nonfatal) compared with those who ate them less than once a week. Those who ate nuts one to four times a week had a 27 percent reduction in heart attacks.

Why nutritionists are nutty about nuts

Why would nuts—which contain more than 50 percent fat—work in your heart's favor? There are five reasons to explain why nuts are heart-friendly.

Good fats

Nuts carry a mix of heart-protecting monounsaturated and polyunsaturated oils in their natural state. For example, the fat in almonds is composed of 68 percent monounsaturated fat and 22 percent polyunsaturated (making a total of 90 percent unsaturated), which leaves only a mere 10 percent saturated fat. Apart from coconut, all nuts contain very little saturated fat and no cholesterol (see table on page 50).

Vitamin E

Nuts are rich in this antioxidant, which works to keep your LDL cholesterol from being oxidized and deposited on artery walls.

Fiber

Nuts carry fiber, which helps lower cholesterol while keeping your bowels regular.

Arginine

Nuts are high in this amino acid, which is converted to nitric oxide in the body. Nitric oxide helps blood vessels dilate and, like aspirin, reduces the stickiness of the platelets in the bloodstream.

Minerals

Nuts are rich in minerals like magnesium, copper, potassium, and selenium, which help protect the heart.

To date, walnuts, almonds, and macadamias have been the three nuts studied for the benefits they can bring to your health, but there's no reason to believe other nuts won't work the same way. In clinical trials, all three have lowered both total cholesterol and LDL when eaten in place of some of the usual fatty foods and spreads—not in addition to them.

Aim for:

➥ A handful of nuts a day (30–50 g), unsalted, raw, or roasted

Nut	Fat content (%)
Mainly monounsaturated	
Cashews	47
Peanuts	49
Almonds	53
Pistachios	54
Pecans	65
Macadamias	75
Mainly polyunsaturated	
Chestnuts	3
Hazelnuts	36
Sesame seeds	49
Walnuts	52
Pine nuts	54
Brazil nuts	62
Mainly saturated	
Coconut, desiccated	62

Ways with nuts

❥ The best way to consume nuts is lightly roasted but not salted.

❥ Add oomph to salads and stir-fries by tossing in a few toasted nuts before serving. You get a lot of flavor for only a small amount of fat!

❥ Substitute nuts instead of potato chips, corn chips, and similar salty snacks. They have similar levels of fat, but it's a healthier fat than the saturated type. Nuts are easy to nibble on—and overeat. If you need to lose weight and find it hard to stop at just a handful, it's probably easier to use nuts to enhance your cooking rather than eating them as a snack.

❥ Make up a fruit-and-nut mix to nibble on. Try my recipe on page 191.

❥ Add nuts to muffins and breads. Or scatter them on top before baking for a crunchy topping.

Whole grains

There have always been good reasons to eat whole grains like grainy breads, bran cereals, whole grain cereals, brown rice, and dark rye breads. And now your heart's health is another one.

Because they contain all parts of the grain, including the highly nutritious germ and the outer bran layers with their nutrient-rich aleurone layer, whole grain foods give us a number of powerful, heart-friendly compounds:

❥ Fiber

❥ Resistant starch ("invisible" fiber)

❥ Folate, thiamin, niacin, and lesser amounts of other B vitamins

❥ Vitamin E and related substances known as toco-trienols

❥ Trace minerals such as magnesium, iron, zinc, phosphorus, selenium

❥ Phytochemicals (that work as antioxidants) like flavonoids, isoflavones, lignans, saponins, and phytates

For example, among the different grains, linseed stands out as a source of omega-3 fatty acids; oats and barley contain beta-glucan, a type of soluble fiber; wheat bran is known for its lignans, which share similar properties to soy isoflavones (see page 47).

The large Nurses' Health Study that's been underway in the U.S. since 1984 has reported that whole grains are protective against heart disease. Specifically, out of more than 75,000 women ages 38 to 63, those with the highest intake of whole grain foods were 30 percent less likely to die of heart disease than those who ate the least. This held true even after the researchers adjusted for smoking, body weight, alcohol, vitamin E use, aspirin use, and types of fats consumed.

Why? The researchers noted that the benefits couldn't be fully explained by grain nutrients like fiber, folate, and vitamin E.

Perhaps another explanation is that many (but not all) whole grains have a type of carbohydrate that is slowly released into the bloodstream, so they don't demand as much of the body's insulin and only slightly raise blood sugar levels when they are eaten. These have been called low-GI foods, meaning Glycemic Index (see pages 53–54). Eating foods with low GI values has an important impact on heart health, as it seems to prevent the resistance or insensitivity to the insulin that is a central part of the Metabolic Syndrome (see page 15). So the more slowly absorbed whole grain foods and legumes you eat, the more you'll make your body sensitive to insulin, which is better for your heart.

Aim for:

❥ 6 servings of breads, cereals, pasta, or rice (or more) a day, with at least 3 of these being whole grain

Tips for increasing your intake of whole grains

- Look for breakfast cereals that are made from bran (Kellogg's All-Bran) or that say whole wheat or psyllium on the label.
- Have coarse rolled oats for breakfast. In summer, make muesli to have over fresh fruit.
- Munch your way through a good natural muesli.
- Add a sprinkle of oat bran or raw psyllium to your usual cereal.
- Swap your white bread for a heavy whole grain or dark rye bread. Good choices are Wonder Stone Ground 100% Whole Wheat, Mestemacher Three Grain, and Alvarado St. Sprouted Sourdough. The chewier, the better.
- Snack on bread in the form of whole grain rolls, toast, English muffins, or pita bread.
- If you own a bread maker, add grains to your home-made loaves. Try linseed, kibbled (cracked) wheat, polenta (cornmeal), rolled oats, or barley meal.
- When baking muffins or cakes at home, throw in a handful of kibbled wheat, wheat bran, or oat bran with the flour, or use whole grain flour.
- Aim to have a pasta meal every day. Although it's not whole grain, it's slowly absorbed. Also look for soy wheat pasta.
- Switch to brown rice.

The GI factor

The Glycemic Index, or GI, is a measure of how a carbohydrate food affects blood sugar. Foods that raise blood sugar quickly have a high GI, while those that raise it slowly have a low GI.

There's More to Heart Health than Cholesterol

This is influenced by:
- The type of starch in the carbohydrate (and the size of its granules)
- Whether the food is processed or cooked
- Whether there is any fat accompanying the carbohydrate
- Whether there is any fiber accompanying the carbohydrate.

Food	GI factor
Low GI	
Rice bran	19
Grapefruit	25
Pearl barley, boiled	25
Soy drink	31
Yogurt, low-fat fruit	33
Soy and linseed bread	36
Apple/pear	38
Pasta (all types)	32–55
Bran cereal	42
Pears, canned	44
Apple muffin	44
Raisin bread	47
Baked beans	48
Moderate GI	
Popcorn	55
Sweet corn	55
Honey	58
Rice (basmati)	58–59
Muesli bar	61
Sugar (sucrose)	65
Shredded Wheat	61–69
Bread, whole grain	69

High GI

Bread, white	70
Corn chips	72
Sports drink	73–78
Pumpkin, boiled	75
Jelly beans	80
Rice, white	85
Potato (boiled, mashed, or baked)	88–93
Parsnip, boiled	97
Glucose	100

Figures reproduced with permission from *The GI Factor: The Glucose Revolution*, by J. Brand Miller, K. Foster Powell, and S. Colagiuri (Hodder & Stoughton, 1996).

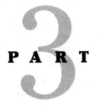

PART

Putting Food

to Work

for You

HOW TO CHANGE YOUR DIET

All the theory in the world is no help unless you know how to put it into practice! This section shows you—clearly and simply—how you can put food to work for your health. I've made it as practical as possible so you can translate the principles into shopping lists, delicious but healthy meals, efficient menus, and easy recipe ideas. To begin with, I've listed the first steps you need to take when embarking on a new way of eating.

STARTING OUT:
5 WAYS TO MAKE YOUR KITCHEN
HEART-FRIENDLY

1.

Stock up on the basics

Milk

Head off to your supermarket and buy a carton of low-fat or skim milk for cereal, milkshakes, smoothies, tea, and coffee. This is especially important if you like lots of milk. You don't have to buy skim milk, as any of the low-fat milks have around the same fat content but with much better flavor—they're not such a big drop in taste. If dairy is a problem for you or you're trying to eat more soy, opt for a low-fat soy drink instead.

Oil

Keep a couple of different oils in the kitchen for cooking and salad dressings. Choose canola or olive oil for everyday cooking, extra-virgin olive oil for salads, sesame or peanut oils if you like Asian cookery, and fragrant gourmet oils such as walnut or macadamia for special salads. Invest in a can of no-stick oil spray.

Margarine/spread

Stop using butter! Instead, buy a tub of soft margarine or spread (preferably one made from olive or canola oils). If you already use a spread, consider one with plant stanol esters (for example, Benecol) to help bring down cholesterol. If you don't like spread, you could consider olive oil, hummus, or spreading some avocado on your bread.

Condiments

These are good to add flavor to lean meats, fish, and sandwiches. I suggest a jar of mustard (Dijon or grainy), a good fruit chutney, a bottle of sodium-reduced soy sauce, a bottle of Worcestershire sauce, and barbecue sauce or horseradish—depending on your preferences.

Bottled pasta sauces/dinner sauces

These are ideal for quick meals. Generally tomato-based sauces are low in fat, but you can check the Nutrition Information Panel on the label—choose ones with less than 5 g of fat per 100 g.

2.

Check what you have in the cupboard

Make sure you have:
- Suitable cereals—made from oats, barley, psyllium, or whole grains
- Bread—whole grain
- Pasta
- Rice—brown or long-grain
- Noodles
- Baked beans and/or creamed corn
- Canned three-bean mix or chickpeas for salads
- Canned kidney or soybeans to stretch out casseroles or meat dishes
- Cans of tuna and salmon
- Salad dressing or oil and vinegar
- Mayonnaise or creamy dressing—buy fat-free or low-fat
- Rye crispbread, plain crackers, and rice cakes
- Popcorn and pretzels for snacks

3.

Check what you have in the fridge

- Milk or soy drink (low-fat) or low-fat milk with stanol esters
- Yogurt, low-fat—plain and fruit—or low-fat yogurt with stanol esters
- Cottage cheese/ricotta cheese
- Lean meat for barbecue or grilling

- Chicken breast fillets
- Fish (fillets, cutlets, or whole)
- Vegetarian dinner option, e.g. soy burgers or tofu burgers

4.

Check what you have in the freezer

- Frozen vegetables—peas, corn, beans, spinach
- Phyllo pastry
- Bread—keep a loaf or some rolls frozen
- Frozen yogurt or low-fat ice cream for dessert
- Fish fillets
- Oven-bake french fries (8 percent fat or less)

5.

Fresh produce

- Potatoes
- Onions
- Garlic
- Selection of fresh vegetables—carrots, broccoli, tomatoes, mixed lettuce, and cucumber are good to start
- Selection of fresh fruit for snacks or light desserts, depending on what's in season—bananas, apples or pears, oranges, grapes, kiwifruit, pineapple, passionfruit
- Fresh herbs for adding flavor—coriander and basil are great (you can grow your own)

THE HEALTHY HEART
SHOPPING GUIDE

Good foods to stock up on

When you're shopping, look for these healthier items to put in your cart. They are all relatively low in fat or saturated fat and will give your diet a bonus of good health. If in doubt, look for products displaying the American Heart Association's heart-check mark. Foods with this symbol are evaluated to ensure they meet the criteria for saturated fat and cholesterol for healthy people over the age of two.

Vegetables

- Any type of fresh or frozen vegetable
- Canned vegetables—look for reduced-sodium or no-added-salt varieties
- Herbs, fresh or dried

Avoid herb salts, herb meat tenderizers, and herb pastes, which often contain salt.

Beans

- Fresh, canned, or dried
- Baked beans—reduced-sodium type
- Three-bean mix
- Kidney beans
- Chickpeas
- Cannellini beans
- Soybeans
- Soy foods such as tofu, tempeh, soy burgers, soy nuggets
- Lentils

Fruit

- Fresh, frozen, or dried—any type
- Canned—buy fruit canned in light syrup or natural juice. It's handy to have at home if you run out of fresh fruit.

Juices count as fruit, but they are deficient in fiber and easy to overconsume. This makes them a diet trap if you're watching your weight. Remember, it takes two or three pieces of whole fruit to make a glass of juice. So limit yourself to one 8-oz glass of juice a day, and dilute it with water and/or ice cubes.

Breads and crispbread

Best choices are whole grain types (now considered protective for the heart):

- Mixed grain, soy and linseed, 100% stone-ground whole wheat
- Whole grain Lebanese bread, whole grain lavash
- Wheat or rye crispbread
- Rice cakes, corn cakes

White bread is still a nutritious low-fat food but lacks the fiber and extra nutrients of whole grain.

Flours and grains

Best choices are whole grain types:

- Brown rice, barley, bulghur wheat
- Use whole grain and soy flours for baking (can replace up to half the white flour in recipes for muffins and cakes)

White rice, couscous, polenta, semolina and pearl barley, while not whole grain, are nevertheless all low-fat foods and are fine in your diet from time to time.

Pasta and noodles

- Pasta (spaghetti, macaroni, fettucine, lasagna, etc.)—all types, both dried and fresh
- Ravioli, tortellini, gnocchi, cannelloni
- Soy pasta
- Noodles—plain types, both dried and fresh

Avoid instant noodles or crisp noodle snacks, which are first fried and contain around 20 percent fat, generally palm oil. The flavor packets with instant noodles are also very high in salt.

Breakfast cereals

Best choices for your heart are cereals made from oats, barley, rye, or psyllium, as they contain more soluble fiber (see page 38):

- Untoasted muesli
- Rolled oats, minute oats
- Bran cereals like Multi-Bran Chex

Other healthy choices:
- Soy cereals
- Whole wheat cereals like Kellogg's Frosted Mini-Wheats
- Fruit and flake cereals like Post Raisin Bran

All cereals (except toasted muesli) are low in fat and are suitable. Corn Flakes, Special K, and similar cereals, while not whole grain, are nevertheless low-fat foods and are fine in your diet occasionally.

Oat bran, rice bran, barley bran, and raw psyllium can be found at supermarkets or health food stores and can be sprinkled over your favorite cereal.

Meat

- All lean meats, trimmed of visible fat—beef, lamb, veal, pork, venison, rabbit
- Chicken, no skin—breast, breast fillet, strips, and trimmed thighs are best choices
- Turkey, duck—no skin.

Organ meats are lean, but some are high in cholesterol. Liver and kidneys have the most cholesterol and should be limited to twice a week.

Fish and seafood

- Fresh, frozen, and smoked
- Canned fish—salmon, mackerel, tuna, sardines (opt for types canned in springwater or tomato and no-added-salt or reduced-sodium); flavored canned tuna is a good choice
- Frozen fish fillets—look for reduced-fat types
- Oysters, shrimp, crab, scallops, mussels, calamari (squid), lobster, abalone—grilled, barbecued, broiled, or steamed, not deep-fried or in a creamy sauce
- Oily fish—such as Atlantic salmon, smoked salmon, fresh tuna, trout, herring, mackerel, blue eye cod—are higher in omega-3s than other fish.

Limit calamari and shrimp to twice a week if your cholesterol is high or you're just starting out on your cholesterol-lowering program.

Milks

- Skim, low-fat, or reduced-fat milk or low-fat milk with stanol esters
- Soy milk—choose low-fat types

- Flavored low-fat milk
- Canned evaporated skim milk
- Buttermilk

Cheese

- Opt for reduced-fat cheeses, but remember that these have only 25 percent less fat—they are still relatively high in fat, so use sparingly
- Mozzarella and Swiss cheeses are lower in fat and salt than other types
- Cottage cheese
- Low-fat ricotta
- Parmesan—use a little shaved and sprinkled on top for flavor

Yogurts and dairy desserts

- Low-fat and diet yogurts, plain or fruit, or low-fat yogurt with stanol esters
- Low-fat custard
- Low-fat dairy desserts
- Reduced-fat ice cream—only as an occasional treat
- Tofu ice cream, soy ice cream—look for reduced-fat

Eggs

- Omega-enriched if available, or regular.

Limit of 4 eggs a week if your blood cholesterol is high.

Nuts

Best choices are unsalted nuts, either raw or roasted:
- Walnuts, almonds, macadamias, pecans, hazelnuts, cashews, Brazil nuts, peanuts, pine nuts, pistachios, chestnuts

- Peanut butter—choose no-added-salt or reduced-sodium types
- Nut butters

Use coconut and desiccated coconut sparingly. For Thai dishes and curries, use canned light coconut milk or half regular coconut milk and half stock.

Seeds

All types, unsalted:
- Linseed (flaxseed), sunflower, pumpkin seeds, sesame, tahini (sesame seed paste), poppy seeds

Spreads

- The best choice if you have high cholesterol is a stanol ester spread (e.g., Benecol or Take Charge). Otherwise, buy any monounsaturated spread (made from canola or olive oil) or polyunsaturated spread (sunflower, soybean) that is reduced-sodium. Avoid butter and dairy blends.
- Light cream cheese spread (use sparingly)
- Mayonnaise (use sparingly); low-fat mayonnaise or mayonnaise with stanol esters
- Avocado
- Hummus

Oils

- Any oil is fine, except for coconut oil or palm oil. Canola oil and olive oil are good general oils; extra-virgin has a stronger flavor.
- No-stick oil spray (for spraying baking tins and frying pans)

Blended vegetable oil is a mixture of several different oils. If it is labeled as polyunsaturated, it is a good choice.

Note that "lite" or "light" oils are lighter in flavor than normal oils, not lower in fat.

Sauces and dressings

Most sauces are high in salt (even reduced-sodium soy sauce), so they should be used sparingly. But they add flavor and make fat-trimmed meats and vegetables taste delicious, so they are a useful addition to your kitchen.

- Sauces—reduced-sodium soy, chili, Tabasco, Worcestershire, fish, oyster, teriyaki, hoi sin, plum, barbecue
- Marinades
- Pesto
- Salad dressings—regular, no-oil and low-fat dressings with stanol esters
- Vinegar—wine, balsamic, cider

Snacks

- Air-popped popcorn (not microwaveable which has 18 percent added fat)
- Pretzels, preferably unsalted
- Breakfast bars

Sweets

- Fruit roll-ups—fat-free but not a substitute for fresh fruit
- Licorice

All chocolate is high in fat, including light chocolate. Some chocolate lovers defend it, saying that its main saturated fatty acid is stearic acid, which does not raise blood cholesterol. However, chocolate is calorie-dense and very easy to overeat. If you can stop at one or two pieces, it's fine. Otherwise, it's better not to buy any at all.

Chewing gum, mints, jellies, jubes, and lollipops are all fat-free but add calories to your diet.

Pastry

> ❥ Phyllo pastry sheets—brush every second sheet lightly with oil, or use orange juice

Miscellaneous

> ❥ Tomato pasta sauces
> ❥ Tomato paste
> ❥ Stock
> ❥ Jarred minced garlic, ginger, chili, coriander
> ❥ Mustards, relishes, chutneys
> ❥ Spices and dried herbs—oregano, mixed herbs, Italian herbs, cumin, five spice, lemon grass, turmeric, tarragon, thyme, dill seeds, sage, fennel, bay leaves, paprika, cinnamon, cloves, nutmeg

FOOD LABELS: HOW THEY CAN HELP YOU

When shopping, you can learn a lot about the fat content of a product from the label.

1. Check the Nutrition Information Panel

Look at the "Percent Daily Value" for fat (based on a 2,000-calorie diet). If it's 8 percent, for example, then a serving of that food supplies you with 8 percent of your recommended fat intake for the day. If a food is advertised as 97 percent fat-free, this simply means it contains 3 percent fat, with water, protein, carbohydrate, fiber, vitamins, and minerals making up the other 97 percent.

Words to watch out for

It's even more important to check the fat content if you see wording on the label like:

- NO CHOLESTEROL
- CHOLESTEROL-FREE
- LIGHT
- REDUCED-FAT
- BAKED NOT FRIED

No cholesterol or cholesterol-free

Even though the food has no cholesterol, it can still be high in saturated fat and should be avoided. This applies to foods like potato chips, corn chips, salty snack foods, pies, pastries, biscuits, sauces, and doughnuts. Remember that NO CHOLESTEROL does not mean NO FAT.

Lite or light

Can apply to a food's texture, flavor, or salt or alcohol content, not necessarily that it is low in fat. Light potato chips are thinly sliced and lightly salted, but still have the same amount of fat as normal chips; light olive oil has a blander flavor but the same fat content as regular olive oil. But light cheese does have less fat than regular cheese, as does light margarine (spread), light cream cheese, and light sour cream. If in doubt, always read the Nutrition Information Panel.

Reduced-fat

Seen on reduced-fat milks, cheese, ice creams, mayonnaise, sour cream, and dairy desserts. Contains less fat than regular products, but may not necessarily be low in fat, i.e., 3 percent or less. Usually such foods have 25–30 percent less fat, so they still taste good and help you save on fat. But you can't eat them as if they were fat-free foods.

Vegetable oil

Don't be fooled into thinking this means the product contains an unsaturated vegetable oil such as canola or olive oil. If one of these oils is used, the label will tell you.

The words "vegetable oil" usually mean palm oil, a tropical oil with 50 percent saturated fat, which is cheap and commonly used by the food industry to fry fast foods and make snack foods. Like all oils, it has no cholesterol but is high in saturated fat and is not recommended for your heart.

A word about hydrogenated fats: During food processing, fats may undergo a chemical process known as hydrogenation. This changes a liquid oil, naturally high in unsaturated fat, to a more solid and more saturated form. Many commercial foods contain hydrogenated or partially hydrogenated vegetable oils.

Hydrogenated fats may be used in the American Heart Association diet if they contain liquid vegetable oil as the first ingredient and no more than 2 g of saturated fat per tablespoon.

Baked not fried

These words often appear on snack foods and implies that the food is low in fat. For some snacks, like pretzels, this is true. But for others, like baked potato chips, it means they are *lower* in fat (around 25 percent) than a fried snack would be but not necessarily *low* in fat. Check the Nutrition Information Panel for the grams of fat per serving.

2. Check the list of ingredients

Ingredients are listed in descending order by weight, so the largest ingredient will appear first on the list, followed by the next, and so on—except for water, which is usually listed at the end as WATER ADDED.

If some type of fat appears as the first or second ingredient, you can assume the product is fairly high in fat and should be eaten sparingly, as most commercial fats are derived from beef tallow or palm oil and thus are saturated.

Fat can be listed as:
- VEGETABLE SHORTENING
- VEGETABLE OIL
- BUTTER
- TRIGLYCERIDES
- COCONUT

Below is an example of a typical label from a cereal bar with a Nutrition Information Panel.

What the Nutrition Information Panel tells you:

- One bar contains only 4 grams of fat, which is fairly low (6 percent of your day's total).
- Only 1 of the 4 g of fat is saturated.
- One bar gives you 2 g of fiber, the same as from a slice of whole grain bread.
- There is no cholesterol present, but that's because there are no sources of animal foods present.

Should you buy it? It's a pretty good choice, being fairly low in fat with good fiber. If you're on a very low fat diet (say 40 g per day), then it would account for 10 percent of your day's fat intake, so ask yourself if you really want it.

Nutrition Facts

Serving Size: 1.3oz/40g (1 Bar)
Servings per container: 4

Amount per serving
Calories: 155
Calories from fat: 36

	% Daily Value*
Total Fat 4g	6%
Saturated Fat 1g	5%
Cholesterol 0 mg	0%
Sodium 5 mg	0.2%
Total Carbohydrate 29g	10%
Dietary Fibre 2g	8%
Sugars 15g	
Protein 2g	

Vitamin A 0% • Vitamin C 0% • Calcium 1% • Iron 3%

*Percent Daily Values are based on a 2,000 calorie diet. Your daily values may be higher or lower depending on your calorie needs.

	Calories:	2,000	2,500
Total Fat	Less than	65g	80g
Saturated Fat	Less than	20g	25g
Cholesterol	Less than	300mg	300mg
Sodium	Less than	2,400mg	2,400mg
Total Carbohydrate		300g	375
Dietary Fibre		25g	30g

Calories per gram:
Fat 9: • Carbohydrate: 4 • Protein: 4

THE HEALTHY HEART IN THE KITCHEN

Ten tips to cook healthier

1. Don't fry meat or chicken in oil, margarine, or butter. Rather, try to broil, roast on a rack, steam, barbecue, or microwave. Try wrapping in foil and baking or barbecuing.
2. When doing a stir-fry in a wok, don't pour lots of oil in. Simply drizzle in a small amount, just enough to stop the food from sticking, or brush or spray a film of oil over the bottom. Stir-fry in stock for a change of pace.
3. Always trim any visible fat from meat, and remove skin and fat from chicken. At the supermarket, look for lean meat with the least amount of fat or marbling.
4. Try not to eat sausages or luncheon meats (unless labeled lean). They are high in saturated fats and cholesterol.
5. Invest in a nonstick frying pan, and simply brush or spray with a little oil for browning. An inexpensive frying pan often works as well as a more costly one, and you can replace it when it gets too "used" on the surface.
6. Cook soups and curries a day ahead, and chill. Any fat will rise to the surface and can be easily skimmed off once it solidifies.
7. If you have time, marinate lean cuts of meat and chicken in wine, fat-free sauces, garlic, mustard, or bottled oil-free marinades. This tenderizes lean meats and imparts a richer flavor.
8. Experiment with vegetarian recipes using firm tofu, canned or dried beans, lentils, or some of the new soy-based dinners. If you're a big meat eater, replace half the meat with canned chickpeas or soybeans.
9. Try adapting some of your existing recipes for cakes or pies to be made with less margarine or oil.
10. If a recipe calls for sour cream, use plain unflavored low-fat yogurt thickened with a little cornstarch.

MODIFYING YOUR RECIPES
TO HELP YOUR HEART

Copy and pin to your refrigerator.

Where your recipe calls for:	Instead use:
Cream	Use canned evaporated low-fat milk mixed with cornstarch
Sour cream	Try yogurt mixed with a little cornstarch
Pastry	Substitute phyllo, spraying between every second sheet; use only a top crust
Oil	Halve the quantity; cook in a non-stick wok or pan; use cooking spray, or brush on oil rather than pouring it on
Lots of meat in casseroles or curries	Halve the meat, add drained canned beans; serve smaller portions on pasta, noodles, couscous, or basmati rice (slow-absorbing carbohydrate foods)
Melted cheese topping	Halve the quantity of cheese, and mix with bread crumbs, rolled oats, or crushed corn flakes; use less cheese by substituting a more strongly flavored one, like Parmesan
Salt	Omit, especially if the dish contains salty ingredients like soy sauce, stock, or bacon; use plenty of fresh herbs, chili, garlic, lemon peel, ginger, and curry powder to add flavor instead

Desserts	Enjoy fresh fruit; add dried fruit and oats to recipes; serve with low-fat custard, low-fat ice cream, or yogurt; try gelato or fruit sorbet in summer
Salad dressings	Use vinegar or lemon juice (their acidity helps to slow down the absorption of carbohydrates)

Kitchen equipment
to make your meals healthier

It's worth investing in these kitchen pieces if you don't already own them, so you can cook with less fat.

Must have:
- Nonstick pan
- Wok
- Charn (wok utensil)
- Electric grill
- Vertical grill

Optional:
- Popcorn maker (for fat-free popcorn)
- Bread maker

HEALTHY HEART MENUS
TO GET YOU STARTED

All of the following menus are low in saturated fat and high in heart protectors. Choose one that suits your situation and your food preferences, and use it as a guide to plan your meals (see pages 127–194 for menu recipes*).

MENU NO. 1:
If you need to lose body fat

If you need to shed body fat, here is one way of eating that's also good for your heart. It gives you plenty of heart protectors like vegetables, fruit, fish, garlic, and soy without overloading you with calories. It's essential that you do some exercise as well (preferably every day) which will greatly help your efforts.

This day's meal plan provides about 40 g fat, of which 12 g are saturated, 215 mg cholesterol, 44 g fiber, 1,910 mg sodium, and 1,900 calories.

Breakfast
Wedge of cantaloupe or papaya
1.5 oz bowl of psyllium cereal or untoasted muesli
with low-fat milk
OPTION: Top with 3 tablespoons
low-fat vanilla yogurt or a small sliced banana
Tea, juice, low-fat milk, or soy milk

Lunch
Crusty whole grain roll lightly spread with mayonnaise,
margarine, or avocado filled with 3.5 oz drained canned salmon or tuna
and lettuce, cucumber, grated carrot, sprouts, and Spanish onion
OPTION: Add a small can of three-bean salad,
drained and drizzled with vinaigrette as a side dish
7-oz bowl of fresh fruit salad

Dinner
6–8 oz char-broiled steak topped with Tomato Basil Salsa*
6 oz garlic mashed potato
Steamed broccoli or green beans—large serving
7 oz low-fat berry yogurt topped with 3.5 oz fresh blueberries
or strawberries plus 2 tablespoons puréed berries
OPTION: If you're really hungry, start with a bowl of soup.
Try vegetable, minestrone, noodle, or tomato.
Don't add sour cream—add evaporated skim milk instead.

Snacks

Choose 3 snacks to have any time between meals or after dinner:
1 Banana Bran Muffin*
Super Smoothie*
2 slices toasted whole grain bread lightly spread
with stanol ester spread (e.g. Benecol)

MENU NO. 2:
When your weight's fine

This day's meal plan is low in saturated fat, but with less restriction on healthy fats and calories than the first. It's designed for someone who doesn't need to shed body fat. It also comes with the added bonus of plenty of heart protectors.

This menu provides 80 g fat, of which 13 g are saturated, 130 mg cholesterol, 54 g fiber, 2,070 mg sodium, and 2,420 calories.

Breakfast
5–6 soft prunes
3.5-oz can baked beans or creamed corn
with 2 slices whole grain toast spread
with stanol ester spread (e.g. Benecol)
Tea, juice, low-fat milk, or soy milk

Lunch
4 oz fettucine or spaghetti tossed with tomatoes,
soybeans or cannellini beans, bell peppers, olives, and basil
Tossed green side salad with The Best Salad Dressing*
OPTION: Add some diced skinless chicken to the pasta if desired
6-oz container of low-fat mango fruit yogurt

Dinner
6–8 oz fish fillet cooked in a pan sprayed with oil
and a sprinkle of chives
Baby potatoes roasted with garlic and rosemary
Steamed green beans or broccoli
Steamed carrots

OPTION: Multigrain roll spread with stanol ester spread (e.g. Benecol)
OPTION: Glass of wine
1 serving Fresh Plum and Ricotta Strudel*
with 2 scoops low-fat vanilla ice cream

Snacks

Choose 3 snacks to have anytime between meals or after dinner:
1.5 oz unsalted roasted nuts (walnuts, almonds, or macadamias)
Cereal bar
1 portion of Fruit and Nut Snack Pack*
8 oz of vegetable soup with 2 rye crackers
1 fresh pear or apple
1 Banana Bran Muffin*

MENU NO. 3:
Mediterranean-style menu

A meal plan for anyone who loves Italian, Greek, or Spanish cuisines. It's based around olive oil, tomatoes, pasta, garlic, seafood, salads, and vegetables—plenty of heart protection here.

This day's meal plan provides 100 g fat, of which 13 g are saturated, 145 mg cholesterol, 48 g fiber, 2,140 mg sodium, and 2,470 calories.

Breakfast

1 cup diced canteloupe or fresh peach slices
4 grilled tomato halves with basil, extra-virgin olive oil drizzled on top
2 slices thick toasted whole grain bread
Tea, juice, or soy milk

Lunch

Large bowl of fettucine or macaroni tossed with roasted bell pepper, roasted eggplant, tomatoes, walnuts, and 3.5 oz can of tuna
Tossed green salad with oil and vinegar dressing
Mineral water or juice

Dinner
Chunky minestrone soup with whole grain roll
6–8 oz fish fillet cooked in a nonstick pan with thick basil pesto
Baked pumpkin wedges
Green beans or zucchini drizzled with olive oil and topped with toasted almonds
2 scoops gelato with canteloupe wedge and grapes
Option: Glass of wine

Snacks
Choose 3 or 4 depending on your appetite:
2 apricots, 2 plums, or a bunch of grapes
1 wedge of canteloupe
1 thick slice of bread with fresh tomato slices and basil leaves
1.5 oz walnuts or almonds
1.5 oz of fresh ricotta drizzled with honey
Raw vegetable sticks with cottage cheese and herbs

MENU NO. 4:
If you're vegetarian

While vegetarian diets are generally healthy eating, not all vegetarian meals are necessarily low in saturated fat. Recipes with lots of melted cheese toppings, thick creamy sauces, coconut-laced curries, and deep-fried items spell disaster for someone overweight or with high cholesterol. Here's one way to eat vegetarian that's good for the heart. Remember that the essentials of a balanced vegetarian diet—lots of vegetables, salads, beans, lentils, and whole grains—will benefit you.

This day's meal plan provides 90 g fat, of which 19 g are saturated, 60 mg cholesterol, 41 g fiber, 2,160 mg sodium, and 2,390 calories.

Breakfast
1 orange
4-oz bowl of rolled oats with brown sugar and low-fat milk
or soy milk or 1.5 oz bowl of untoasted muesli

1 slice whole grain toast, spread with 1 tablespoon peanut butter

Juice, soy milk, or herbal tea

Lunch

Mixed lettuces, cucumber, roasted red bell pepper, celery, sprouts, and tomatoes topped with a small can of three-bean mix and 3.5 oz cottage cheese, drizzled with The Best Salad Dressing*

Large whole grain roll with stanol ester spread or hummus

Strawberry smoothie made with 1 glass low-fat milk or soy milk, honey, and ½ cup fresh strawberries

Dinner

Tofu and vegetable stir-fry made with 2 oz firm tofu slices, marinated, and 2 cups sliced vegetables such as onion, celery, bell pepper, snow peas, carrot, bok choy, or beans

1 cup noodles

6 oz low-fat berry yogurt topped with 4 oz fresh blueberries or strawberries plus 2 tablespoons puréed berries

OPTION: If you're really hungry, start with a bowl of soup. Try pumpkin, vegetable, minestrone, noodle, or tomato. Don't add sour cream—add evaporated skim milk instead.

Snacks

Choose 3 snacks a day to have at anytime:

1 Banana Bran Muffin* with stanol ester spread

1 slice whole grain bread spread with crunchy peanut butter

2 or 3 rice cakes topped with spread, sliced banana, and honey

1.5 oz roasted cashews or peanuts

1 pear, peach, or other fresh fruit

MENU NO. 5:
Asian style

A meal plan for those who like Asian cuisine. It's low in fat overall but will fill you up with lots of rice, noodles, vegetables, and
fish. Just go easy with the salty soy and fish sauces.

This day's meal plan provides 45 g fat, of which 10 are saturated, 250 mg cholesterol, 25 g fiber, 600 mg sodium, and 2,150
calories.

Breakfast

Plate of assorted fruit—pineapple, papaya,
canteloupe, peach, strawberries

1.5 oz bowl of psyllium cereal or whole grain cereal
with low-fat soy milk or low-fat milk

Option: Top with 3 tablespoons low-fat vanilla yogurt
or a small sliced banana

Green tea, jasmine tea, or fruit juice

Lunch

Bowl of thin noodles stir-fried with mixed vegetables such as
cabbage or Asian greens, bell pepper, green onion

Option: Add 2 oz sliced or diced chicken breast or tofu cubes

Green tea or jasmine tea

Dinner

150 g White Fish with Sesame and Ginger*

Stir-fried bok choy (or other green vegetable)

1 cup steamed rice

Fresh mango half or pineapple wedge

Snacks

Choose 3 or 4 depending on your appetite:

1 skewer chicken or lean pork pieces, marinated

1 glass fruit puree/juice

1 oz rice crackers

8 oz bowl of steamed rice

Large bowl of noodles and stock

MORE IDEAS
FOR HEALTHY HEART MEALS

Breakfast ideas

Filling breakfasts-on-the-go that are low in saturated fat and high in fiber:

1 cup bran cereal with 2 tablespoons grapes or raisins
1 small banana, sliced
1–2 tablespoons oat bran
½ cup low-fat milk

1 large apple, grated with the skin, mixed with 7 oz of low-fat plain yogurt and 2 tablespoons one-minute oats

3–4 prunes
1 cup bran or psyllium-based cereal
½ cup low-fat milk

½ cup natural muesli
½ cup low-fat milk topped with 3 tablespoons low-fat apricot yogurt

1½ cups cooked rolled oats (made with half water, half low-fat milk)
Sprinkle of brown sugar or honey
1 slice whole grain toast
1 tablespoon peanut butter

½ grapefruit
½ whole grain muffin, toasted, topped with tomato slices and a slice of reduced-fat Cheddar cheese, grilled

Glass of orange juice
4 oz baked beans
2 slices whole grain toast

2 toasted whole grain muffin halves
½ cup cottage cheese
Tomato slices

Smoothie made with:
1 cup skim or low-fat milk
1 small banana, sliced
1 tablespoon honey or sugar
1–2 tablespoons oat bran or wheat germ

½ baked apple
½ carton natural yogurt topped with cinnamon
1 whole grain roll, toasted
1 teaspoon soft margarine or stanol ester spread

Lunch ideas

Takeout might be handy, but most items are notoriously high in saturated fat and salt—a definite no-no for your heart. However, today more and more sandwich shops, sushi bars, and even fast-food outlets are selling healthier offerings. Whether you pack your own lunch or buy it, here are ideas for quick lunches for busy bodies.

Tuna on bread
1 slice of thick whole grain bread
4 oz can tuna, drained
Lettuce, sliced celery, grated carrot, and thinly sliced Spanish onion

Thai beef salad
Thin slices of lean roast beef (4 oz)
Chili sauce
Tomato and cucumber wedges
Assorted lettuce leaves and fresh coriander
½ cup fine noodles

There's More to Heart Health than Cholesterol

Whole grain pita (or lavash flatbread) filled with 3–4 oz cold cooked
chicken, shredded lettuce, and tabbouleh
Bunch of grapes or cherries

Salmon pasta salad
5-oz bowl of cooked macaroni
4-oz can salmon, drained
Strips of roasted red bell pepper
Cucumber
Basil leaves

4-oz can baked beans
1 slice thick toasted whole grain bread
1 fresh pear

Hamburger made with lean ground beef, soft whole grain roll,
tomato, lettuce, cucumber
6-oz carton low-fat strawberry yogurt

Risotto made with 4 oz chicken pieces, 2 tablespoons walnuts,
½ cup sliced mushrooms
Tossed salad

Bowl of vegetable soup
Tuna and lettuce sandwich on whole grain bread
2 or 3 dried apricots

Minestrone or thick vegetable soup
2 slices thick rye bread toast topped with 3 or 4 canned sardines

Salmon and bean salad
4 oz salmon mixed with ½ cup of white beans, chopped scallions,
red pepper, sliced or grated carrot, chopped parsley
Vinaigrette dressing
Slice of rye bread, light spread

Tuna and butter bean salad
4-oz can tuna
½ cup canned butter beans, drained
Macaroni or pasta spirals
Mixed lettuce leaves

Bean and vegetable soup
Whole grain roll
1 slice reduced-fat cheese

Dinners and main meal ideas

Light and easy meals in under 30 minutes.

Fillet of perch (6–8 oz), grilled or baked, brushed with a ginger-soy marinade
1 cup thin noodles, boiled
Stir-fry mixed vegetables

Fillet of white fish, barbecued and topped with fresh chili, lime juice, and coriander sprigs
2 or 3 char-broiled sweet potato slices
Char-broiled zucchini halves

Salmon cutlet or steak (6–8 oz) topped with lemon juice and fresh dill
½ cup mashed potatoes
Tossed green salad with The Best Salad Dressing*

Snapper fillet (6–8 oz), char-broiled or barbecued
1 baked potato
1 large serving ratatouille

6-oz can of tuna in springwater, drained, tossed with
1 cup cooked pasta spirals or penne and topped with diced fresh tomato, basil leaves, and olives
Tossed green salad with vinaigrette

There's More to Heart Health than Cholesterol

2 chicken kebabs topped with lemon yogurt sauce
½ cup steamed rice
Large serving of steamed green beans or broccoli
Large serving of carrots

1 chicken breast fillet, marinated in pesto and slow-baked
½ cup couscous
Large serving of zucchini and asparagus

Roast chicken with light gravy
1 baked potato
1 piece baked pumpkin
½ baked parsnip
Large serving of steamed broccoli

Fillet or rump steak (5 oz), barbecued or grilled with
cracked black pepper and Dijon mustard
1 serving of baby new potatoes
1 cob corn
1 serving of broccoli or brussels sprouts

Beef and snow pea curry
¾ cup steamed long-grain rice
Cucumber salad
Chutney

Stir-fried beef strips with bell pepper, bok choy,
and celery in a honey-soy sauce
½ cup noodles or rice

Warm beef salad
3–4 beef strips, stir-fried with onion, bell pepper, and zucchini
1–2 cups mixed lettuce leaves drizzled with The Best Salad Dressing*

2 or 3 lamb cutlets, char-broiled, topped with Tomato Basil Salsa*
3–4 boiled new potatoes
Large serving of green beans

2 lamb and vegetable kebabs with Asian-style sauce
½ cup boiled thin noodles

4 oz pork fillet, marinated in Worcestershire sauce, orange juice,
and wine and baked until just cooked
1 baked potato
Large serving of spinach
Large serving of carrots

1 thin veal steak, sautéed with lemon and garlic
1 cup oven-baked potato and herb wedges
2 grilled tomato halves

Stir-fry of tofu, asparagus, and Asian greens*
½ cup boiled noodles

1 large baked potato filled with ½ cup chili bean mixture
Tossed green salad with vinaigrette dressing

Fettucine with napoletana (tomato, garlic, and herb) sauce
Tossed salad of mixed lettuces, cucumber, and sprouts
Drizzle of oil and vinegar dressing

Snack ideas

Between-meal snacks are the downfall of most of us. Our modern world is filled with snacks that beckon—chips from vending machines, chocolate bars at the mini-mart, popcorn at the movies, candy at the supermarket checkout, and cookies stashed in our desk or locker at work.

Snacking in itself is not bad—it does have certain nutritional benefits such as spreading the glucose load or firing up the body's metabolism. To achieve this, the type of snacks we choose is critical. You don't have to eliminate everything you love, but you shouldn't indulge in excess—meaning once or twice a week, not every day.

There's More to Heart Health than Cholesterol

If you're serious about dropping your cholesterol, here are some lower-fat healthy alternatives. Some you'll have to plan ahead to take with you, some you can buy.

- Fresh roll with peanut butter and grapes
- Snack pack of almonds or walnuts with dates and raisins
- Toasted whole grain muffin spread with cottage cheese and tomato slices
- 3–4 crackers with reduced-fat cheese or peanut butter
- Rice cakes topped with thick jam
- Cereal bar—low-fat
- Handful (1–2 oz) of peanuts, almonds, walnuts, or macadamias
- Small pack (1 oz) of pretzels
- Bowl of air-popped popcorn
- Date scone with a little spread
- Plain scone with light cream cheese and jam or honey
- Low-fat banana or blueberry muffin
- Raisin bread, fresh or toasted, spread with a little stanol ester spread (e.g. Benecol)
- Handful of breakfast cereal
- Raw carrot sticks (or celery or zucchini strips) with hummus or low-fat dip
- Fresh fruit salad
- Fresh pear or peach
- Bunch of frozen grapes
- Carton of fresh blueberries or strawberries
- Kiwifruit, cut in half and scooped out with a spoon
- Carton of low-fat fruit yogurt
- Carton (8 oz) flavored low-fat milk
- Gelato or fruit ice
- Fruit juice or lemonade ice pop

WHAT YOU NEED TO KNOW
ABOUT ALCOHOL, COFFEE, AND SALT

Alcohol and the heart

Modest consumption of alcohol—wine, beer, or spirits—is good for the heart. Red wine has stolen the limelight with the realization that the French, whose diet oozes saturated fat thanks to their butter, cream, pâté, and pastries, have one of the world's lowest rates of heart disease. (In fact, they are second lowest after Japan.) The explanation scientists came up with for this so-called "French Paradox" is the red wine that the French love to sip with their meals.

There's ample research to show that wine has a positive effect on cholesterol. In a 1995 study, a group of 17 healthy men with no cholesterol problems consumed their usual meals with two glasses of wine every day for two weeks. After the two weeks, those who drank red wine showed a 72 percent drop in the "readiness" of their LDL cholesterol to undergo oxidation, an early step in heart disease. But those drinking white wine had no such decrease.

In another study of almost 1,200 people in California, those who consumed moderate alcohol were found to have 30 percent less risk of having a coronary event than those who drank no alcohol.

Nutritionists have identified the polyphenols in red wine as the key compounds in benefiting the heart, as they act as antioxidants and slow down the oxidation of LDL cholesterol. These natural grape-derived substances, such as quercetin and resveratrol, give red wine its characteristic sharpness or bite. They are mainly found in the skins and stalks of grapes, so are much more prevalent in red than in white wine. White wine has about one-tenth the amount of these phenols as red, which explains its lesser effect.

But don't forget that the alcohol from any drink—wine, beer, spirits, or liqueur—can also boost levels of good HDL cholesterol, which is another mechanism by which moderate drinking lowers heart disease rates.

Aim for:
- ❥ No more than 2 glasses a day (for men)
- ❥ No more than 1 glass a day (for women)
- ❥ Ensure you have some days free of alcohol

Tea and coffee

Numerous studies have tried to lay blame on caffeine as a cause of heart disease, but over the years no clear-cut solid evidence has emerged. Moderate caffeine intake, for instance 3–6 cups of instant coffee a day (equivalent to 1–2 cups of freshly brewed coffee), does not seem to raise cholesterol or blood pressure or cause heart attacks. Coffee drinkers often appear to have more heart disease than non-coffee drinkers because many of them also smoke, which is the real danger.

How you brew your coffee may be important, however. Research has found that boiled, Turkish, Greek, Scandinavian, and plunger coffee (French press) can send cholesterol levels up. Any sediment-rich brew that is made without a filter contains tiny particles of ground coffee (called fines) and oil droplets that can raise cholesterol and triglycerides. It's not the caffeine but two diterpene substances called kahweol and cafestol that are the cause. Espresso and cappuccino have a similar, although smaller, effect.

If you drink your coffee drip-filtered through paper or percolated, it contains negligible amounts of diterpenes and so doesn't cause any concern.

Tea drinking, on the other hand, appears to be good for your heart. Several large studies have reported a link between tea and heart disease—the more tea you drink, the less likely you are to suffer heart problems.

Both green and black tea contain a number of flavonoids, which act as antioxidants and have been linked to reductions in heart disease. Green tea's catechins, notably the much-studied epigallocatechin gallate (EGCG), have been suggested as a prime reason for the low death rate from heart problems in Japan and China. The addition of milk to ordinary tea does not affect the absorption of the flavonoids into the body.

According to one study published in the *American Journal of Epidemiology* in 1999, people who drank one or more cups of tea a day had a 44 percent lower risk of a myocardial infarction (heart attack) compared with people who drank no tea. The researchers investigated the coffee- as well as tea-drinking habits of 340 case-control pairs from the Boston, Massachusetts, area. For coffee, they found no link to heart attack even though they started their investigation suspecting they would find coffee bad for the heart.

It makes good sense to switch from coffee to tea as part of a heart-healthy diet. Tea has one-third to one-half the caffeine of coffee, which is another advantage for those who are sensitive to the stimulating effects of too much caffeine.

Aim for:
- 3–4 cups of tea a day
- a maximum of 3 cups instant coffee, which is equivalent to 1 cup espresso or cappuccino.

Salt

Cutting back on salt is important for heart health because it can keep hypertension (high blood pressure) at bay, which is one of the key risk factors for heart disease and stroke. Although hotly debated among nutritionists, I feel you really do need to consume less salt. There are many advantages and no disadvantages.

Some people can consume as much salt as they like with no ill effects, while others are what scientists now call "salt sensitive" (estimated to be around 15 percent of the population). In other words, if they eat a lot of salt, their blood pressure will rise. If they cut back, their blood pressure drops back to normal.

If high blood pressure runs in your family, it's likely that you are salt sensitive. And research shows that salt reduction helps if your blood pressure is high or you're overweight or over 50 (as we age, salt affects us more).

Other dietary factors that help lower blood pressure are:
- Losing body fat
- Drinking less alcohol
- Getting more of three beneficial minerals—potassium, magnesium, and calcium. A high intake of these appears to counteract sodium
- Increasing your intake of omega-3s (see page 36).

Aim for:
- Consuming less than 1,000 mg sodium a day (ideal) but with a maximum of 2,300 mg sodium a day.

Where's the salt coming from?

Commercial foods	75%
Salt used in cooking and added at the table	15%
Natural sodium in foods (found in fish, meat, milk, cocoa powder, and some vegetables, notably celery and spinach)	10%

Tip

Chemically, salt is sodium chloride. It is the sodium part that causes health problems. A teaspoon of salt contains 2,000 mg sodium, so you should be eating less than half a teaspoon a day total.

Seven ways to make a difference in your salt intake

1. Buy reduced-sodium and no-added-salt foods whenever you can. This will have the biggest impact on your total salt intake, as salt is a common ingredient in so many commercial foods. In fact, these foods supply around 75 percent of all the sodium we eat.

    Key foods to choose in reduced-sodium form are bread, margarine, reduced-fat cheeses, breakfast cereals, canned vegetables, sauces and peanut butter, even though many of these do not taste salty.
2. Cut out salty-tasting foods like anchovies, salted pretzels, potato chips, and olives. These perpetuate a liking for saltiness and create a noticeable thirst, which explains why they are traditionally served with drinks.
3. Gradually use less and less salt at the table (some sneaky people even block up some of the holes in the salt shaker). However, while worthwhile for reeducating your palate, this will reduce your total sodium by only 15 percent.
4. Potassium chloride, a salt substitute, can help during the first few weeks. It is white, crystalline, and can be shaken on food like salt. However, some people detect an unpleasant metallic aftertaste. Most people discontinue it after a few weeks because they lose the desire for saltiness. Anyone with kidney problems should check with their doctor first, as excess potassium can spell trouble for compromised kidneys.
5. Gradually reduce the amount of salt you use in cooking.
6. Initially, cook recipes with half the normal quantity of salt, reducing it as you progress. Do not add salt if you use salty ingredients, such as bacon, soy sauce, bottled sauces, Parmesan cheese, etc. Use unsalted margarine or oil for baking cakes.
7. Add flavor with herbs, spices, curry powder, and aromatic ingredients like lemon juice, orange peel, mustard powder and wine. Use plenty of chili, onions, garlic, and shallots.

Take care to read the list of ingredients on the labels of things like marinades, meat tenderizer, and curry powders—some have salt that will hinder your efforts.

FAST FOOD CHOICES

What to choose when eating out and ordering fast food

As a rule, most fast food is not a heart healthy choice. Portions tend to be over-generous, even more so with the trend to "another 20 percent free" offers and jumbo sizes for very little extra money. It's generally high in fat and calories and is excessively salty. These two factors alone make fast food a fat-inducing way of eating. And because the whole atmosphere in fast-food restaurants is geared towards eating FAST, eating in your car, or eating while you walk, it promotes eating too much food, too quickly—a real trap for anyone with a weight problem.

But in addition, if you're watching your fats and cholesterol, most fast food is high in the wrong sort of fats. Anything that's deep-fried ends up being high in saturated fat, because the commercial frying fats are saturated. There are moves towards healthier oils for deep-frying that I applaud, but their use is still fairly limited.

Even if fast food is not deep-fried, it still usually high in "hidden" fats, as is the case with soft hamburger buns, pizza, or nachos. This is because fat has many useful functions in fast food—it keeps baked goods like buns or pizza crust soft and moist; it makes corn chips crisp; and it creates an aroma in anything served hot.

Here are the best choices if you're out and about and the only choice is fast food.

Sushi/California rolls

Light and almost fat-free, these seaweed-wrapped rice rolls, filled with tuna, cucumber, or avocado, are a godsend. Just go easy with the salty soy sauce. Numerous sushi bars are now popping up in city locations.

Noodle soups

Some stir-fried noodles with meat and vegetables can be greasy, but the clear soups with noodles from Japanese or Asian food bars are generally a great choice—warming, filling, and with very little fat. To increase the protein, order yours with tofu or fish pieces.

Burgers

Look for plain burgers served in an old-fashioned burger joint where the bun is toasted and you get tomato, lettuce, and onion with the meat patty. Steer clear of double or triple burgers from the chains, which stack on the fat and calories. You don't need the ones with bacon or cheese.

Chicken burger

If it's a skin-free grilled piece of chicken, this is a good choice that appears from time to time on the menu of fast-food chains. If it's crumbed or a patty, it's similar in fat to a hamburger. Don't be fooled into thinking that because chicken is white meat it is therefore lighter.

Skin-free/marinated chicken pieces

Many new chicken outlets have appeared recently with lower-fat chicken options, which is great news. Go for these grilled or barbecued chicken pieces, and add a salad, coleslaw, and roll to make a balanced meal.

Steak sandwiches

Generally lean and fairly filling. Same comments as for hamburgers. Ask for lettuce, tomato, and onion to bulk the sandwich up and fill you up—but not cheese.

Baked potatoes

Hot and hearty for a cold winter's day. No fat in the potato or its skin, but watch those toppings. Say no to cheese and sour cream with chives. Instead go for salsa.

Wraps

A wrap filled with ham, chicken, tuna, or roast beef and lots of veggies makes a good lunch or snack for busy workers. Try not to buy ones with loads of mayonnaise or cheese.

Burritos

Soft burritos filled with beans, avocado, and veggies are the best low-fat choice at Mexican restaurants.

Asian

Every Asian food bar does things differently, so it helps to try one out and see how they compare.

- Chinese—stir-fry pork or beef with vegetables, stir-fry chicken with vegetables, corn and chicken soup, clear soup with noodles, san choy bau
- Thai—Thai beef salad, beef or chicken satays, dry curries (without a lot of coconut milk) all served with jasmine rice
- Vietnamese—clear hot and sour soup (pho) with chicken or beef, chicken vermicelli soup, seafood and vegetable combination served with rice or thin noodles

❥ Japanese—noodles with fish, chicken or pork; soups with noodles and vegetables; sashimi (raw tuna or salmon); bento boxes

WHAT YOU CAN DO ABOUT VISIBLE AND HIDDEN FATS

1. Visible fat—be sparing with the fat that you can see

Oils

Oils add healthy fat to your diet and boost your intake of unsaturated fats. But we don't need huge amounts. Aim for 1 or 2 tablespoons of oil a day for cooking and over salads or with crusty bread. Try to get out of the habit of frying or roasting food in oil. You don't need heaps of oil to fry—just enough to stop food from sticking.

❥ Good choices: monounsaturates such as olive oil and canola oil
❥ Other choices: polyunsaturates like sunflower oil and safflower oil (check the label for the word polyunsaturated)
❥ Use an oil spray for oiling frying pans, woks, and muffin trays.

Spreads

❥ Forget butter. For bread, just scrape on a little margarine. If you're using a stanol ester spread, you can be more generous (see page 30).
❥ Low-fat or fat-free mayonnaise is a good choice—any fat is usually unsaturated. Low-fat mayonnaise is lower in fat than margarine.
❥ Other good choices are tahini, avocado, and hummus.

- When spreading peanut butter, no need to first spread the bread with margarine. The peanut butter, at just over 50 percent fat, has enough fat content to moisten the bread.
- Light cream cheese is another alternative for bread, bagels, and scones. At only 14 percent fat, it's lower than margarine or mayonnaise—but the catch is it's saturated fat. Still, when spread lightly on a slice of bread, this translates into less than 2 g of fat.

Meat and chicken

- Trim all visible fat off meat, and remove skin from chicken
- Don't buy meat that is marbled (has fatty streaks throughout).
- If all the fat is removed, red meat has a similar fat and calorie content similar to white meat such as veal and chicken.
- If your weight is a problem, aim for small- to medium-size portions—around 5 or 6 oz.

HEART MYTH

WHAT YOU'VE HEARD: Red meat is much worse for the heart than white meat.

FACT: Red meat can be as lean and healthy as white meat (chicken, veal, pork, fish), provided you buy lean cuts and trim off any visible fat. Leaner cuts include loin and round cuts.

2. Hidden fats—a trap for the unwary

Many foods contain a lot of fat, but you can't see it because it's part of the food's makeup.

Snacks

- Steer clear of chips and other salty snacks, even if labeled "lite" (this usually means lightly salted or thinly sliced, not lower in fat). All such snacks are fried in palm oil, which is largely saturated fat or hydrogenated oils.
- If you need a snack, opt for pretzels (unfortunately high in salt), or pop your own popcorn using a little oil to prevent sticking. Don't use microwave popcorn, as it is high in fat.
- Take care with snacks that say they are "baked not fried." They still have some fat added to the dough before baking, even though they are not deep-fried. They are lower in fat than fried snacks, but are not low-fat.
- Choose puffed rice or rice cakes
- Go easy on processed snack items made with hydrogenated or partially hydrogenated vegetable oil.

Fast food

Fast food is generally high in saturated fats due to the use of palm oil or beef tallow for deep frying.

Dairy foods

- Switch to low-fat (1–2 percent fat) or skim (less than 0.5 percent fat) milk.
- Buy low-fat or fat-free yogurt.
- Use cottage cheese and ricotta for toppings and to make dips.

- Look for reduced-fat cheeses when shopping. Most of these have one-third less fat than regular Cheddar cheese (27 instead of 33 percent), meaning that they are lower in fat but not necessarily low-fat. (Low-fat foods by law must have 3 percent fat or less.) So reduced-fat cheeses are helpful, but be sparing about how much you eat.
- Stop using cream and sour cream (35 percent fat). Light versions have half the fat of regular varieties—but they're still high in fat.

HEART MYTH

WHAT YOU'VE HEARD: A Healthy Heart diet should be low in fat.

FACT: Healthy Heart diets come in many forms. The Mediterranean Diet, which embraces the traditional cuisines of southern Italy, Greece, and Crete, is HIGH in fat—but the fat is largely monounsaturated from olive oil. The Asian Diet, typified by the diet of Japan, China, and Southeast Asia, is low in fat and high in carbohydrates. What both these different eating patterns have in common is that they are low in SATURATED fat, the bad food fat linked to heart disease (see sample menus 3 and 5 on pages 80 and 83).

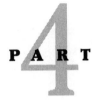

PART

4

When Diet

Isn't Enough

EXTRA HELP FOR YOUR HEART

If you have high cholesterol or high triglycerides, your doctor will usually begin treating you with diet therapy—a Healthy Heart diet as detailed in this book. You will also have to commit to regular exercise and lead a healthier lifestyle. You will be asked to have your blood fats remeasured after 6 weeks or 2 months.

If you're diligent and committed, you'll find that the changes in your diet and lifestyle should bring about a drop in the cholesterol and/or triglyceride levels. For some people, however, even though they follow the steps carefully, it will not be enough. Here then are the options that your doctor will discuss with you when you need a stronger program.

MEDICATIONS

Medications for the heart are usually needed for long periods, perhaps even for a lifetime. Like all drugs, they have side effects, so it's important that you continue following a healthy diet and exercising. You'll then be able to take the lowest dosage to achieve results, which will minimize the possibility of side effects.

The four medications described here are the most commonly prescribed. Discuss them with your doctor or pharmacist so you understand exactly how they act in the body, why you need them, and how side effects will be monitored.

1. Statins

If you have high LDL cholesterol, and diet and exercise haven't helped, your doctor will probably start you on a course of one of the statin drugs such as:

- Atorvastatin (Lipitor)
- Simvastatin (Lipex, Zocor)
- Pravastatin (Pravachol)
- Cerivastatin (Lipolay)
- Fluvastatin (Vastin, Lescol)

These medications work by inhibiting an enzyme known as HMG-CoA reductase, which is responsible for manufacturing cholesterol. When the drug reduces the manufacture of cholesterol by organs such as the liver, the body makes up the deficit by taking the harmful LDL out of the bloodstream.

Studies testing the statin drugs have reported a 20–60 percent lowering of LDL levels, a reduction in triglycerides, and a modest rise in levels of HDL.

Their side effects are infrequent and mild—in a small number of people, statins may irritate the muscles or the liver—but generally they are well tolerated.

2. Bile acid resins

One of the earliest treatments for high cholesterol, resins such as cholestyramine (Questran) or colestipol (Colestid) act by "mopping up" bile acids in the intestine which are then eliminated in the feces. They do not enter the bloodstream, because they are not absorbed from the intestine.

Although effective, many people find them hard to keep taking due to their unpalatability and the common digestive disturbances that are linked to them, like constipation, gas, bloating, stomach upset, nausea, and heartburn.

Lately, smaller doses of these drugs have often been combined with a statin; this combination produces a greater benefit with less gastric upset.

3. Nicotinic acid

Nicotinic acid is a B vitamin, also known as niacin. At high doses of 1,500–3,000 mg a day (hundreds of times the recommended daily intake from food), it has proven very effective at lowering LDL cholesterol by 30–40 percent, lowering triglycerides by 20–50 percent and raising HDL by 15–35 percent.

It probably enhances the effectiveness of other drugs such as the statins, but there is a theoretical risk that it could increase the likelihood of their producing side effects. In practice, however, this is an infrequent occurrence, so the combination is becoming more popular.

At these high doses, nicotinic acid is acting as a drug. And like drugs, it can have side effects. The most common is flushing, due to the dilating of blood vessels of the face, which is sometimes accompanied by itchy skin, rashes, stomach upset, and headache. It can also raise blood sugar and lead to gout.

Slow-release niacin was developed to minimize the facial flushing but some formulations have been associated with an impairment in liver function. Even though nicotinic acid is cheap and available without a prescription, don't take it yourself. It should be used only under your doctor's supervision so the effects can be monitored with blood tests.

Nicotinamide, another form of niacin, does not lower cholesterol and should not be used in its place.

4. Aspirin

One of the world's most widely used medicines, aspirin taken daily in low dose form can lower the risk of heart attack and stroke by limiting the ability of the platelets in the blood to stick together and form a clot. Dosage is usually 75–150 mg a day.

Aspirin has been publicized for its ability to reduce the likelihood of a second heart attack and death in people with existing heart disease. Use it in conjunction with other measures like controlling cholesterol and high blood pressure.

Aspirin too can have side effects and won't suit everybody, so it's essential to discuss it with your doctor.

SUPPLEMENTS FOR THE HEART

Check with your doctor before taking these, especially if you are taking any of the above four medications regularly.

Fish oil

Fish oil capsules, with their powerful omega-3 fatty acids, are a safe and usually effective treatment for anyone with high triglyceride levels. They have no effect on cholesterol.

In addition, fish oil capsules can thin the blood and steady the heartbeat, thus reducing irregular or chaotic heartbeats that can trigger an attack. In some cases, fish oil lowers blood pressure as well.

The American Heart Association suggests an intake of 2 g of omega-3 fatty acids a day (equivalent to 6 g of fish oil or about 6 capsules) to lower triglycerides.

Fish oil has few adverse effects. But because it decreases your blood's ability to clot, two groups of people who shouldn't take fish oil capsules are those with a bleeding disorder or those taking anticoagulants such as warfarin.

Vitamin E

Vitamin E (also called alpha-tocopherol) is an antioxidant vitamin. Originally, researchers felt this fat-soluble vitamin could keep the heart healthy by:

❥ Stopping LDL from being oxidized
❥ Promoting blood flow
❥ Stopping blood cells from clumping, an action similar
  to aspirin and fish oil

Unfortunately, the results of research trials on vitamin E have been mixed. The early ones were quite favorable—a 1996 U.S. study of more than 34,000 older women in good health who participated in the Iowa Women's Health Study reported that women who ate the most foods rich in vitamin E cut their risk of dying from heart disease by more than half. Another study from Cambridge University (the CHAOS study) found that vitamin E pills reduced the risk of heart attack by one-third.

On the other hand, an Italian GISSI prevention study using 150-mg vitamin E tablets contradicted these results. And a relatively large trial spanning 4–6 years—the HOPE trial—showed vitamin E was of no benefit in reducing heart problems in patients at high risk. So there is no clear advice on vitamin E at this point.

Unlike other antioxidants, the quantities of vitamin E needed are high, over and above what can be obtained via diet. The trials that showed positive benefits used vitamin E at 400 International Units (IU) a day or higher, which is impossible to obtain from food alone (The Daily Value for E is 30 IU).

To get even half this amount, you would have to swallow spoonfuls of vegetable oil or bowlfuls of nuts, hardly feasible if you're trying to shed weight.

If you do supplement, look for a brand with 500 IU (or 335 mg) per tablet—any more is not necessary, although the chance of toxic side effects is low. Multivitamins generally carry less than 10 IU, while ACE antioxidant supplements usually have 100 IU, both of which are insufficient. However, ACE antioxidant supplements do offer a combination of vitamin E with water-soluble antioxidants such as vitamin C, which may work better than vitamin E alone.

Garlic

The ancient Egyptians, Vikings, and Chinese all believed in garlic's power to keep the heart strong, but until recently there was not enough convincing evidence to confirm or deny this long-standing reputation.

Garlic, in the form of dried garlic powder, garlic oil, or aged extract, has been tested in many studies in both animals and people to see if it can lower blood cholesterol levels. Typically, patients have taken 600–900 mg of standardized garlic powder (a high dose—equivalent to 10–20 g of fresh garlic or 2–4 cloves) every day for 8–24 weeks.

Three meta-analyses (overviews) have been published since 1994. The latest, which looked at 13 well-conducted double-blind garlic trials, has concluded that garlic powder does lower cholesterol when compared to a placebo (a dummy pill) but the effect is only modest.

When combined, the 13 trials achieved a modest drop in cholesterol but not strong enough to replace any medications your doctor may prescribe.

The authors reported that only 13 of 39 trials met the inclusion criteria for analysis. This means two-thirds were excluded, which may have an important effect on the conclusions. While the analysis found that overall garlic powder did reduce cholesterol more than a placebo, the six studies considered of higher quality showed no reduction in cholesterol levels when taking garlic.

There's also evidence showing that garlic can keep the arteries more flexible and elastic as well as thin the blood and promote circulation.

So while the evidence is weak for garlic capsules, there's no reason to stop using garlic in your cooking. It contains a variety of natural antioxidants and strong-smelling sulphur compounds that can help your overall health and may protect your cholesterol (in a small way) against harmful free radicals.

Lecithin

Over the years, numerous claims have been made for lecithin, including that it lowers cholesterol.

Lecithin is rich in an oily substance called phospholipid, which has phosphorus as a key ingredient. It is made by the body in our liver and is a component of bile (where it keeps gallstones from forming). It aids in the digestion and transport of fats—this is probably where the belief in its cholesterol-lowering powers originally arose.

As a supplement, you can take it as granules or capsules. And you can obtain it from food—it's found in egg yolks, wheat germ, liver, soy, legumes, and grains such as maize. Unlike vitamins or minerals, lecithin and phospholipids are not essential nutrients. However, lecithin does contain choline and inositol, two compounds often associated with the B vitamins.

Some lecithin is high in polyunsaturated fats, which accounts for early reports that it could lower cholesterol. It is expensive, however, and you could get these fats much more cheaply from polyunsaturated oils or nuts.

Although few analyses are available, lecithin is probably rich in vitamin E, which accounts for its ability to protect polyunsaturated fats from oxygen attack. Two tablespoons of lecithin granules supply 10 g of fat and 80 calories. For most people, lecithin is of limited value.

Co-enzyme Q10

Co-enzyme Q10 (also called ubiquinone) is sometimes prescribed by natural practitioners for patients with angina or congestive heart failure. It is also claimed to offset the muscle irritation that can accompany the statin drugs, although evidence is lacking to date.

Co-enzyme Q10 is a natural substance widely distributed in foods, with the richest sources being oily fish (sardines, mackerel), lean meat, soybeans, nuts, and oils. It is an essential component of the mitochondria—the energy powerhouses of the cells—and is needed when they convert fuel into energy. This is especially important for heart muscle, which is one of the most metabolically active tissues in the body. Co-enzyme Q10 works as an antioxidant but does not lower cholesterol.

Co-enzyme Q10 is also made by our bodies, so supplements only boost what's normally present in us. However, there is some evidence that levels of Co-enzyme Q10 decline with age, so older people may benefit the most from supplementing with it.

At the usual doses of around 100 mg a day, co-enzyme Q10 appears safe, but it would be considered only a small part of an overall treatment plan.

Hawthorn

Hawthorn is a traditional herbal remedy. It appears to work by dilating the coronary blood vessels and increasing blood flow to the heart.

Hawthorn is a white-flowered shrub or small tree with attractive white or pink flowers that bloom in May in Europe, hence its popular name, mayflower. It was widely used in Europe during the late nineteenth century for treating heart problems.

In Germany, France, and Russia hawthorn enjoys official drug status for the treatment of heart ailments. Apparently it has a direct, favorable effect on the heart and can have a noticeable effect in cases of heart damage.

Its active components are pigments called flavonoids and procyanidins. They can lower blood pressure, boost contractions in the heart, and stabilize a rapid heartbeat.

Hawthorn looks to be promising, but its actions have not been proven. While one day it may turn out to be an effective supplement for heart trouble, at present don't take it without a doctor's advice.

Chinese red yeast rice supplement

Red yeast rice is the fermented product of rice on which red yeast (*Monascus purpereus*) has been grown.

Red yeast has a long history in China, where it's used to make rice wine, as a preservative, and for its medicinal qualities. Chinese medical texts note it is prescribed for improving the circulation of the blood.

In China and Japan, red yeast rice is a common food today. Chinese researchers have studied it in both animals and humans and reported that it can reduce cholesterol by 11–32 percent and triglycerides by 12–19 percent.

In the U.S., a dietary supplement (Cholestin) of red yeast rice was recently evaluated for its usefulness for heart patients. The yeast appears to produce a number of chemicals that are very similar to cholesterol-lowering statins or HMG-CoA reductase inhibitors—although the researchers pointed out that these were not present in sufficient quantities to explain the extent of the yeast's cholesterol-lowering effect.

Red yeast rice also contains plant stanol esters, isoflavones, and monounsaturated fats—all elements that protect the heart. At this stage, it's an interesting product, but just how useful it is remains to be proven.

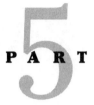

PART 5

Live Your

Lifestyle

A healthy diet works better if you also change your lifestyle—get more exercise, quit smoking, and find ways to deal with the stress of our day-to-day lives.

1. EXERCISE

Regular exercise has many benefits for your heart. It can:

- Raise levels of protective HDL
- Improve your circulation
- Lower blood pressure
- Burn off calories and raise your body's metabolic rate, making weight loss easier
- Make your muscles more receptive to insulin.

Activities that use the large muscles of the body (thighs, trunk, and shoulders) are good forms of exercise; they give your heart and lungs a cardiovascular workout. Some of these are:

- Brisk walking
- Swimming
- Tennis
- Bicycling
- Dancing (ballroom, disco, country)
- Skipping
- Aerobics

The important thing is to find a sport or activity that you like and that fits your schedule—and do it regularly. Even gardening or heavy housework are forms of exercise!

While the standard advice has been to do 20–30 minutes of strenuous aerobic exercise at least three times a week, in recent times more moderate exercise, like walking, has been advocated.

Aim for 30 minutes every day or every second day. It doesn't have to be done in one block—three sessions of 10 minutes can be substituted for one long exercise period. And remember, a little exercise is better than none at all.

2. QUIT SMOKING

If you smoke, take steps today to give up the habit.

According to the American Lung Association, more than 44 million Americans have quit smoking. Many smokers make several attempts before they successfully quit. But it can be done!

Planning ahead seems to make a big difference to your success. Here are the elements of a successful quitting program (most smokers usually include a combination of these strategies):

- Social support from family and friends
- Having a quitting "buddy"
- Attending a course or weekly program for group support
- Counseling
- Stop-smoking aids such as nicotine patches, chewing gum, or inhalers—talk to your pharmacist or doctor
- Tablets to reduce cravings and withdrawal symptoms— you'll need a prescription from your doctor
- Relaxation techniques (hypnotherapy)
- Cutting down gradually
- Going cold turkey
- Using the four D's to deal with cravings (Delay, Deep breath, Drink water, and Do something else).

The American Lung Association's *Freedom from Smoking*® program offers support in the form of guidebooks, videotapes, and audiotapes. The program is now offered online as well; for 24-hour stop-smoking support, log on to www.ffsonline.org. Or call your local Lung Association at 1-800-LUNG-USA.

3. DEAL WITH STRESS

The role of stress in heart disease has been difficult to pin down.

Researchers once divided people into two personality types. Type A people were thought more likely to develop heart disease at an earlier age than their opposites, Type B. The Type A person was highly competitive, aggressive, always driving to achieve goals and a perfectionist. Type B people were more relaxed, easygoing, and unhurried.

However in recent years these two classifications have been shown to be too simplistic. Research is now looking at people who are angry, hostile, aggressive, or depressed. These traits seem more predictive of who will get heart disease than the earlier types.

In the workplace, studies have consistently shown that people in high-stress jobs but with little sense of control (such as bus drivers) have the highest rates of heart attacks. Jobs often perceived as high stress, such as executives or doctors, tend to have the lowest rates of heart attacks, because these professionals have a greater sense of autonomy and control.

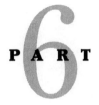

PART

Recipes for

the Healthy

Heart

Here is a collection of healthy recipes that I love to cook, along with ones I've coaxed from friends and colleagues. All are good for the heart, as they are low in saturated fat, low in cholesterol, high in fiber or slowly absorbed carbohydrate, and provide a bonus of heart protectors.

My recipes tend to be quick and easy, so you get maximum result for minimum effort—great for busy lives—but there are many wonderful cookbooks these days that also offer light and fresh recipes that require a little more time. It's worthwhile upgrading your cookbooks as many older ones rely on too much butter or other fattening ingredients and have recipes that are not suited to a heart-healthy style of eating.

USING THE NUTRITION ANALYSIS

Each recipe gives you the quantity of total fat, saturated fat, fiber, sodium, and calories it contains. In addition, I've highlighted those that give you omega-3s, plant stanol esters, antioxidants, folate, soy, nuts, and whole grains, those wonderful heart helpers spelled out in this book.

The recipe analyses are based on the listed ingredients in each recipe. They do not include the serving suggestions such as the rice or bread as accompaniments. Where a range of serving sizes is given (such as Serves 4–6), the analysis has been done on the larger figure.

Fat

The quantity of fat suggested for good health is calculated as a percentage of calories eaten. No more than 30 percent of calories from fat is widely accepted as a figure adults should aim for, which translates to 60–70 g of fat a day for a moderately active person.

Fat-free diets are unnecessary and not compatible with health and growth. Even for a Healthy Heart diet, it is important to eat a bare minimum of 40 g of fat a day; utilize healthy fats from foods such as oils, spreads, nuts, avocados, and seeds. These foods will also boost your unsaturated fats and add valuable heart protectors.

Less than one-third of your total fat should be derived from saturated fat, i.e., 15–25 g of saturated fat a day, depending on your total fat intake. All the recipes concentrate on keeping saturated fat low, generally under 4 g a serving, by following the cooking tips given in Part Three of the book. However, it is impossible to avoid saturated fat entirely, as it is found in all foods, even those classified as monounsaturated or polyunsaturated.

Fiber

Eating at least 30 g of fiber a day is suggested for good health for adults. And since most of us don't even get 20 g, we would do well to increase our fiber intake from vegetables, legumes, whole grains, fruits, and nuts.

For children, a handy rule of thumb to work out how much fiber they should have is their age plus 5. So a 10-year-old should aim for 15 g a day. Most of the recipes here maximize fiber intake, particularly the soluble fiber described in Part Three.

Sodium

A maximum of 2,300 mg of sodium a day is recommended, but most of us consume twice this amount. Most of our salt intake comes from everyday foods such as cheese, deli meats, sauces, breads, canned foods, and spreads. Wherever possible, the recipes suggest reduced-sodium or no-added-salt versions of commercial foods.

Although no salt is added to the recipes, some salt will come from ready-made sauces, stock (although it's easy to make your own salt-free stock), mustard, cheese, bread, and ham. Asian-based recipes, with their reliance on soy, fish, or oyster sauces, tend to be high in salt too. I've used the reduced-sodium versions, but go easy with these, as they are still quite high.

Calories

How many calories you should eat will depend on your age, level of physical activity, body size (larger bodies require more), and sex. Children and teens have greater calorie needs due to the demands of growth, as do women who are pregnant or breast-feeding. The following levels are only approximate but serve as a general guide:

Women	Moderately active	2,000 calories
	Sedentary	1,800 calories
	For fat loss	1,500 calories
Men	Moderately active	2,500 calories
	Sedentary	2,000 calories
	For fat loss	1,800 calories

Cholesterol

Cholesterol values have not been listed because all the recipes are low and well within the suggested daily limit of 200 mg.

Heart protectors

Each recipe has key heart protectors listed in a box at the bottom.

Healthy Heart Factor

Stanol esters	Contains sterol-enriched ingredients, such as milk, yogurt, or dressing
Omega-3s	Provides at least 100 mg (as EPA + DHA) in a serving
Soluble fiber	Contains moderate to rich sources such as psyllium, oats, oat bran, legumes, dried fruit, oranges, apples
Folate	Provides at least 40 micrograms in a serving
Antioxidants	Contains ingredients which are rich sources of antioxidant vitamins and/or phytochemicals (there are no recommended intakes for these yet)
Soy protein	Provides at least 6.25 g in a serving
Nuts	Contains at least 10 g in a serving
Low GI	Carbohydrate foods with a GI less than 50 or made with vinegar or lemon juice–based dressing
Whole grains	Unrefined grains such as brown rice, whole grain flour, barley as the predominant starchy food

Tip: Toasting nuts or seeds

A number of the recipes suggest you add toasted nuts or sesame seeds to a dish.

To toast nuts, place them in a nonstick pan over medium heat. Cook while shaking the pan for 2–3 minutes or until nuts are golden. Take care not to burn them. Nuts can also be toasted in a moderate oven (350°F) in a baking tray for 2 minutes, or until golden. Transfer to a plate immediately, or nuts may burn in the retained heat of the pan.

To toast sesame seeds, toss in a dry frying pan over medium heat for a minute or two, or until golden. Transfer to a plate immediately. Alternatively, microwave on high for 20–30 seconds.

❥ Five Fabulous Ways to Cook Fish ❥

Fish with Cilantro Pesto and Couscous

> **SERVES 4**
> **PREPARATION TIME:** 5 minutes **COOKING TIME:** 10 minutes

Use this flavorsome variation of the usual basil-based pesto to enliven any fish.

4 white fish fillets, such as swordfish or cod (about 1½ lb)
1 cup (8 oz) couscous
2 cups boiling water

Cilantro pesto

2 cups loosely packed cilantro, chopped
¼ cup pine nuts, toasted (see Tip, page 126)
2 tablespoons lemon juice
2 tablespoons olive oil
2 tablespoons Parmesan cheese
freshly ground black pepper

❥ BROIL or barbecue the fish for 5 minutes each side, until the flesh flakes with a fork when gently tested.
❥ COOK couscous in 2 cups boiling water according to directions on packet.
❥ PROCESS cilantro, pine nuts, lemon juice, oil, cheese, and pepper together in a food processor until smooth.
❥ SERVE fish on a bed of couscous, topped with a dollop of pesto. Accompany with steamed sugar snap peas and carrots.

Nutrients per serving
Fat: 23.8 g, Saturated fat: 4.9 g, Fiber: 3.7 g, Sodium: 245 mg, Calories: 438, Good for: omega-3s, folate, antioxidants, nuts

White Fish with Sesame and Ginger

SERVES 4
PREPARATION TIME: 25 minutes (includes marinating)
COOKING TIME: 15 minutes

This Asian-style marinade teams well with chicken or pork fillets too.

If you like ginger, use the higher quantity specified.

4 white fish, ocean perch, or whiting fillets (around 1½ lb)
1 tablespoon finely sliced shallots
2 teaspoons toasted sesame seeds (see Tip, page 126)

Marinade

¼ cup sherry, sweet or dry
2 tablespoons brown sugar
2 tablespoons sesame oil
1 tablespoon reduced-sodium soy sauce
2–4 teaspoons grated fresh ginger
2 cloves garlic, crushed
1 teaspoon lime or lemon juice

❥ PREHEAT oven to 350°F.
❥ PLACE fillets in a single layer in a large shallow dish.
❥ COMBINE all marinade ingredients in a bowl. Pour over fish, turning to coat. Stand for 10–15 minutes (or cover, and refrigerate for up to 4 hours).
❥ TRANSFER fish to a baking dish, reserving marinade. Bake, uncovered, for 12–15 minutes, or until fish flakes easily when tested with a fork.
❥ BOIL marinade in a small saucepan for 3–4 minutes, or until slightly reduced and thickened; pour over fish. Sprinkle with shallots and sesame seeds.
❥ SERVE with steamed rice and green beans.

Nutrients per serving
Fat: 15.6 g, Saturated fat: 3.3 g, Fiber: 0.5 g, Sodium: 348 mg, Calories: 355,
Good for: omega-3s,

Kathleen's Lemon Zest Swordfish

SERVES 4
PREPARATION TIME: 10 minutes **COOKING TIME:** 3 minutes

I learned this yummy recipe from my kids' babysitter, Kathleen, who is not only a talented cook but a fitness fanatic, so everything she cooks is light and healthy.

4 swordfish steaks, about ½" thick (about 1½–2 lb)
2 tablespoons flour
grated rind (zest) of 2 lemons
freshly cracked black pepper
4 lemon wedges
4 sprigs Italian parsley

➤ COAT swordfish lightly in flour, shaking off excess.
➤ SPRINKLE one side with half the lemon zest and half the pepper.
➤ SPRAY a heavy frying pan with oil. Preheat pan before adding swordfish steaks, seasoned side down.
➤ COOK 1 minute on the first side (the zest should slightly char). Sprinkle the top with remaining zest and pepper. Turn fish over. Cover pan with a lid for 1 minute to ensure complete cooking.
➤ SERVE with lemon wedges and parsley garnish. Accompany with green beans or a salad and boiled new potatoes.

VARIATION

• Serve fish with a spoonful of good quality relish.

Nutrients per serving
Fat: 5.4 g, Saturated fat: 2.1 g, Fiber: 0.4 g, Sodium: 166 mg, Calories: 229, Good for: omega-3s

Cod with Mango Salsa

SERVES 4
PREPARATION TIME: 10 minutes **COOKING TIME:** 8 minutes

A simply divine combination for when mangos are in season. Try to choose a mango that's firm or even a little under-ripe, with its skin-tinged green.

olive oil for brushing (or oil spray)
4 cod cutlets (about 1½–2 lb)

Mango salsa
1 mango, peeled, stoned, and chopped
2 tablespoons finely chopped purple Spanish onion
½ red bell pepper, seeds removed and chopped
1 tomato, chopped
1 tablespoon each chopped mint and basil
¼ teaspoon chopped chili pepper, or to taste
juice of ½ lime or lemon
freshly cracked black pepper

➤ HEAT a grill. Brush with a little olive oil.
➤ SEAR fish for 30 seconds each side. Cook for a further 3–4 minutes each side, or until cooked to taste.
➤ COMBINE all ingredients for mango salsa in a bowl.
➤ SERVE with salsa, new potatoes, a mixed leaf salad, and lime wedges.

VARIATION
• If preferred, serve on a bed of baby spinach leaves with crisp, oven-baked potato wedges.

Nutrients per serving
Fat: 5.8 g, Saturated fat: 2.2 g, Fiber: 1.5 g, Sodium: 180 mg, Calories: 254,
Good for: omega-3s, antioxidants, low GI

Barramundi and Snow Pea Stir-fry

SERVES 4
PREPARATION TIME: 10 minutes **COOKING TIME:** 5 minutes

It's unusual to see a fish stir-fry, so I was intrigued by this recipe from the "Great Meal Ideas" recipe program initiated by Coles Supermarkets. I've adapted it a bit, but it remains a quick solution to the problem of what to cook for dinner. You can use any firm-fleshed fish in place of the barramundi.

1 tablespoon peanut oil
1 lb barramundi fillets, cut into 1" pieces
1 cup snow peas, trimmed
1 red bell pepper, seeds removed and sliced
8 oz can sliced water chestnuts, drained
3 shallots, sliced
1 teaspoon grated fresh ginger
8 oz fresh Asian noodles
2 tablespoons reduced-sodium soy sauce
1 tablespoon chicken stock or water
2 tablespoons toasted cashews (see Tip, page 126)
2 tablespoons chopped cilantro

- HEAT oil in a wok or large pan over medium to high heat.
- ADD fish. Stir-fry for 1–2 minutes, until just golden. Remove from wok, and set aside.
- STIR-FRY peas, pepper, water chestnuts, shallots, and ginger for 1–2 minutes, or until peas have turned bright green.
- PLACE noodles in a bowl. Cover with boiling water, and let stand for 1 minute. Drain well.
- RETURN fish to wok with vegetables. Add soy sauce and stock. Cook 1–2 minutes to rewarm fish.
- PLACE noodles in 4 serving bowls. Spoon fish and snow pea stir-fry over top. Garnish with cashews and cilantro. Serve immediately.

Nutrients per serving
Fat: 10.6 g, Saturated fat: 2.4 g, Fiber: 4.1 g, Sodium: 476 mg, Calories: 232, Good for: omega-3s, low GI

❧ Five Things to Do with Canned ❧ Salmon and Tuna

Curried Salmon and Vegetables

SERVES 4
PREPARATION TIME: 15 minutes **COOKING TIME:** 30 minutes

A great way to get your oily fish (rich in omega-3s) and vegetables (high in antioxidants) all in one.

2 teaspoons olive oil
1 onion, finely chopped
1 clove garlic, crushed
1–2 tablespoons mild curry paste or powder
½ cabbage, thinly sliced
2 carrots, grated
1 zucchini, sliced thinly
1 red bell pepper, seeds removed and chopped
3 cups low-fat milk or soy milk
¼ cup plain flour
14-oz can pink salmon, drained and flaked
1 tablespoon lemon juice or vinegar
freshly ground black pepper

❧ HEAT oil in a large saucepan. Sauté onion and garlic until onion is tender. Stir in curry paste. Cook, stirring, for 1 minute.
❧ ADD cabbage, carrots, zucchini, and red bell pepper. Cook, covered, over gentle heat until vegetables are wilted. Shake occasionally to prevent sticking.
❧ BLEND a little milk with the flour to make a smooth paste. Set aside.
❧ POUR remaining milk over vegetable mixture (add a little more if needed to just cover vegetables). Bring to a boil. Remove from heat. Gradually blend in flour paste.

❥ RETURN to heat. Cook, stirring constantly, until mixture boils and thickens. Simmer for 3 minutes. Fold in salmon, lemon juice, and black pepper. Heat gently. Serve with rice or on toast with lemon wedges.

VARIATIONS
- Tuna may be used in place of salmon.
- Increase the spiciness of this dish by adding a dash of chili sauce.
- A mixture of soy and chili sauce is delicious sprinkled over this dish.

Nutrients per serving
Fat: 23.8 g, Saturated fat: 4.9 g, Fiber: 3.7 g, Sodium: 245 mg, Calories: 438,
Good for: omega-3s, folate, antioxidants

Thai Salmon Cakes

> **SERVES 4**
> **PREPARATION TIME:** 15 minutes **COOKING TIME:** 10 minutes

Everyone loves these delicious salmon cakes, and they're quick and easy to make.

2 7-oz cans red or pink salmon
1 onion
3–4 fresh chili peppers or 1 teaspoon chili paste (more if you like food hot)
2 teaspoons peanut oil
4 slices whole grain bread, crusts removed
½ cup chopped fresh cilantro
2 eggs, beaten
1 teaspoon grated lime or lemon rind
flour, for coating
oil spray, for cooking

- ◗ DRAIN salmon well, and remove any silver skin or small bones. Place in a small mixing bowl.
- ◗ PROCESS the onion and chili in a food processor, using short bursts until finely chopped, but not minced (alternatively, you can chop by hand).
- ◗ HEAT the oil in a nonstick frying pan. Cook the onion mixture for 1–2 minutes, or until onion turns transparent.
- ◗ PROCESS the bread and cilantro into crumbs. Add crumbs, onion mixture, egg, and rind to the salmon. Mix well with a fork.
- ◗ SHAPE mixture into 8 flat cakes. If time allows, cover, and refrigerate for 10 minutes before cooking. Coat lightly with flour, shaking off excess.
- ◗ SPRAY pan with oil, and cook salmon cakes over medium heat for 5 minutes on each side.
- ◗ SERVE with steamed rice, lime or lemon wedges, extra cilantro, and chili sauce on the side.

Nutrients per serving
Fat: 14.6 g, Saturated fat: 3.6 g, Fiber: 2.8 g, Sodium: 589 mg, Calories: 274, Good for: omega-3s, folate

Mediterranean Vegetables and Tuna

SERVES 4
PREPARATION TIME: 20 minutes **COOKING TIME:** 5 minutes

Tuna teams nicely with tomatoes, eggplant, red bell pepper, and olive oil—all key ingredients of the heart-winning Mediterranean Diet.

1 bunch asparagus, trimmed and halved
4.5 oz green beans, trimmed and halved
3.5 oz snow peas, trimmed
2 small eggplants, halved
3 oz mushrooms, sliced
6 plum tomatoes, sliced
1 red bell pepper, seeds removed and sliced
16-oz can tuna in springwater, drained and chunked
¼ cup olive oil
1 tablespoon lemon juice
1 tablespoon balsamic vinegar
1 teaspoon brown mustard
1 tablespoon toasted pine nuts (see Tip, page 126)

❥ BLANCH asparagus, beans, and snow peas in boiling water for 1 minute. Refresh in cold water, and drain well.
❥ BROIL eggplant under hot grill for 2 minutes, until golden brown.
❥ COMBINE all prepared vegetables and tuna in a large bowl.
❥ POUR over combined oil, lemon juice, vinegar, and mustard. Toss to combine.
❥ SERVE with couscous or spiral pasta. Sprinkle pine nuts over top.

Nutrients per serving
Fat: 18.2 g, Saturated fat: 2.9 g, Fiber: 6.8 g, Sodium: 204 mg, Calories: 287, Good for: omega-3s, folate, antioxidants

Sweet and Sour Tuna Stir-fry

SERVES 4
PREPARATION TIME: 7 minutes **COOKING TIME:** 10 minutes

If you like sweet 'n' sour but don't want it fried, try this healthier version with pineapple and teriyaki sauce.

2 teaspoons peanut or canola oil
1 onion, sliced
1 clove garlic, crushed
1 zucchini, sliced
1 stalk celery, sliced
1 carrot, sliced
½ cup broccoli florets
½ red bell pepper, seeds removed and sliced
¼ cup pineapple pieces, drained
14 oz can tuna in springwater, drained and chunked
6 snow peas, trimmed and halved
3 oz mushrooms, sliced
¼ cup pineapple juice
¼ cup teriyaki sauce
juice of ½ lemon
fresh cilantro

- **HEAT** oil in a wok or large frying pan. Sauté onion and garlic for 1 minute.
- **TOSS** in zucchini, celery, carrot, broccoli, pepper, and pineapple. Stir-fry for 2–3 minutes.
- **ADD** tuna, snow peas, and mushrooms. Stir-fry for 1 minute.
- **BLEND** in pineapple juice, teriyaki sauce, and lemon. Stir-fry until liquid boils. Cook for 1 minute. Serve with rice or noodles and topped with cilantro.

VARIATIONS
- Grated ginger and shallots may be added.
- If preferred, use fresh tuna. Add with initial vegetables.
- Toss fresh noodles in tuna mixture before serving.

Nutrients per serving
Fat: 2.9 g, Saturated fat: 0.8 g, Fiber: 3.0 g, Sodium: 295 mg, Calories: 136,
Good for: omega-3s, folate, antioxidants

Tuna Vegetable Mornay

> **SERVES 4**
> **PREPARATION TIME:** 10 minutes **COOKING TIME:** 5 minutes

A low-fat variation of an old-fashioned favorite.

2 oz soft margarine or stanol ester spread
1 onion, chopped
4 tablespoons flour
2 cups low-fat milk
14-oz can tuna in springwater, drained
7-oz can corn kernels, drained
1 rib celery, chopped
1 carrot, grated
½ cup reduced-fat grated cheese
2 tablespoons chopped fresh parsley
4–5 button mushrooms, sliced + extra for garnish
1 tablespoon lemon juice
2 cups cooked brown rice

- MELT margarine in a large saucepan. Sauté onion until clear. Stir in flour. Cook for 1 minute. Remove from heat. Gradually stir in milk.
- HEAT, stirring constantly, until sauce boils, thickens, and rolls away from base of pan.
- ADD tuna, corn, celery, carrot, cheese, and parsley. Simmer for 3 minutes. Stir in mushrooms and lemon juice.
- PILE rice on a large platter. Make a well in the center. Spoon tuna mornay into the middle, and sprinkle with extra parsley.

Nutrients per serving
Fat: 14.9 g, Saturated fat: 6.8 g, Fiber: 4.5 g, Sodium: 498 mg, Calories: 476, Good for: omega-3s, folate, whole grains

❧ Five Marvelous Meals ❧ with Lean Meat

Char-grilled Steak with Tomato-Basil Salsa

SERVES 4
PREPARATION TIME: 5 minutes **COOKING TIME:** 5 minutes

This quick salsa also works well on top of pork fillets or a bowl of pasta.

4 fillet or rump steaks (about 1½ lb)
2 corn cobs, cut into rounds

Tomato-basil salsa
2 tomatoes
1 small Spanish onion
½ cup chopped fresh basil or parsley
juice of 1 lemon
cracked black pepper

❧ COOK steaks on a preheated grill that's been sprayed with oil. Cook for 3–4 minutes each side for rare or longer for medium. (The meat should be springy when pushed with tongs—do not pierce with a knife or the juices will run out and it will become tough.)
❧ COOK corn, turning until each side is just browned.
❧ DICE tomatoes and onion finely. Add basil, lemon juice, and pepper. Mix to combine. Serve on steak accompanied by corn, boiled new potatoes, and a mixed leaf salad.

VARIATIONS
• Add 1 small or ½ medium avocado, peeled and finely diced, to the salsa.
• Substitute fresh chopped mint for the basil.

Nutrients per serving
Fat: 5.9 g, Saturated fat: 2.2 g, Fiber: 2.3 g, Sodium: 113 mg, Calories: 289, Good for: folate, antioxidants, low GI, whole grains

Dijon Steak
with Butter Bean Salad

SERVES 4
PREPARATION TIME: 5 minutes **COOKING TIME:** 5 minutes

It's amazing how one simple ingredient like mustard or pepper-corns can turn a basic steak into something with zing—without great effort. This idea also works well with thin veal steaks.

4 small lean fillet or rump steaks
(about 1–½ lb)
½ cup beef stock or water
⅓ cup red wine
2 teaspoons Dijon mustard
2–3 teaspoons drained
green peppercorns (see Note)

Butter bean salad

2 10-oz cans butter beans, rinsed and well-drained
8 oz snow peas, trimmed
8 cherry tomatoes, halved
½ cup basil leaves, torn
2 tablespoons extra virgin olive oil
1 teaspoon Dijon mustard
squeeze of lemon juice
freshly ground black pepper

- TRIM any fat from steak, and cut into individual portions if necessary.
- SPRAY or brush a nonstick frying pan with a little oil. Heat pan over high heat. Sear steaks for 30 seconds on both sides.
- LOWER heat. Cook, covered, for 3–5 minutes, depending on the rareness desired. Remove from pan, and keep warm.
- ADD stock, wine, and mustard to pan. Boil rapidly in pan juices for 1 minute. Add peppercorns. Pour over steaks, and serve with butter bean salad and bread.

➤ FOR salad, combine beans, snow peas, tomatoes, and basil in a small salad bowl. Whisk together oil, mustard, lemon juice, and pepper in a small container. Pour dressing over salad, and toss lightly.

NOTE: Green peppercorns packed in water or vinegar are available in jars or cans at good supermarkets and delicatessens. Be warned—they are hot.

Nutrients per serving
Fat: 15.4 g, Saturated fat: 3.7 g, Fiber: 7.4 g, Sodium: 309 mg, Calories: 311, Good for: folate, antioxidants, low GI

Beef, Corn, and Snow Pea Stir-fry with Sesame Oil

SERVES 4
PREPARATION TIME: 15 minutes **COOKING TIME:** 10 minutes

This is an all-in-one stir-fry that gives you meat plus lots of crisp vegetables, all made delicious with the fragrance of sesame.

1 lb lean beef strips
2 teaspoons peanut or canola oil
1 chili pepper, seeds removed and sliced, or a few drops chili sauce
2 teaspoons sesame oil
1 onion, cut into segments
2 cloves garlic, crushed
1 teaspoon grated fresh ginger
9 oz fresh baby corn, halved
4.5 oz snow peas, trimmed
½ red bell pepper, seeds removed and thinly sliced
1 teaspoon sesame seeds, toasted (see Tip, page 126)

Stir-fry sauce
1 teaspoon cornstarch
½ cup beef stock or water
1 tablespoon reduced-sodium soy sauce

❥ REMOVE any visible fat from beef.
❥ HEAT oil in a wok or deep frying pan. Stir-fry beef and chili pepper in 3 or 4 batches for 3 minutes per batch, until meat just changes color (if you cook too much at once, it stews in its own juice and becomes tough). Remove from wok, and set aside.
❥ HEAT sesame oil in same pan. Stir-fry onion, garlic, and ginger for 1 minute. Add corn, snow peas, and bell pepper, and stir-fry for another 2 minutes. Return cooked meat to wok.
❥ MAKE sauce by blending cornstarch with stock and soy sauce. Pour over meat and vegetables in pan. Cook, stirring, until sauce boils and thickens.

➤ SERVE over steamed brown rice or noodles, sprinkled with sesame seeds.

VARIATION
- If fresh corn is not available, substitute a 15-oz can of baby corn, drained.

Nutrients per serving
Fat: 10.4 g, Saturated fat: 2.5 g, Fiber 3.9 g, Sodium: 478 mg, Calories: 241

Beef, Sweet Potato, and Arugula Stack

SERVES 4
PREPARATION TIME: 5 minutes **COOKING TIME:** 20 minutes

Chefs love serving meals in a stack or "tower" of food, so here's how to do it at home.

2 sweet potatoes, peeled and sliced
4 small fillet steaks (¾–1½ lb)
4 plum tomatoes, halved lengthwise
4 large mushrooms
1 tablespoon olive oil (or use oil spray)
1 bunch arugula
1/4 cup balsamic vinegar
1/4 cup maple syrup

❧ BOIL sweet potatoes until tender. Mash well. Keep warm.
❧ PLACE steaks on a hot grill, brushed or sprayed with oil, or under a broiler. Sear steaks for 30 seconds each side.
❧ DRIZZLE tomatoes and mushrooms with oil. Add to grill.
❧ COOK steaks, tomatoes, and mushrooms for 2–3 minutes each side (or until cooked to taste).
❧ ARRANGE mashed sweet potatoes on 4 serving plates. Top with arugula, steak, tomatoes, and mushrooms.
❧ DRIZZLE with combined vinegar and syrup. Serve with a mixed leaf salad and crusty whole grain bread.

VARIATION
• If sweet potatoes are not available, substitute pumpkin or a mixture of half mashed potato with half mashed parsnip.

Nutrients per serving
Fat: 15.2 g, Saturated fat: 3.6 g, Fiber: 5.5 g, Sodium: 94 mg, Calories: 390, Good for: folate, antioxidants, low GI

Lean Beef Skewers
with Chili Ginger Marinade

SERVES 4
PREPARATION TIME: 10 minutes (includes marinating time)
COOKING TIME: 10 minutes

If you love hot and spicy food, try this Asian-inspired recipe. The active ingredient in chili peppers is known as capsaicin, which is responsible for their heat and may work to boost your body's metabolic rate so you burn off fat a little faster.

1½ lb rump steak
2 tablespoons sweet chili sauce
1 tablespoon reduced-sodium soy sauce
2 teaspoons grated fresh ginger
2 cloves garlic, crushed
pinch of Chinese five-star powder
1 onion, cut and separated into slices
1 red bell pepper, seeds removed and cut into squares
8 bamboo skewers, soaked

- TRIM off any fat from beef. Cut into 1" cubes.
- COMBINE chili sauce, soy sauce, ginger, garlic, and five-star in a shallow bowl. Add beef, turning to combine. Cover, and allow to marinate for 30 minutes (or overnight in the refrigerator).
- THREAD beef, onion slices, and pepper squares onto skewers.
- HEAT a grill. Spray with oil. Cook skewers for 10 minutes, or until browned and tender, turning during cooking.
- SERVE with steamed basmati rice and a mixed leaf salad.

TIP
• Soak bamboo skewers in water for 15–30 minutes before using, to prevent them from burning.

Nutrients per serving
Fat: 5.0 g, Saturated fat: 2.1 g, Fiber: 0.6 g, Sodium: 172 mg, Calories: 236

❧ Five Quick Chicken Ideas ❧

Honey-Mustard Chicken

> **SERVES 4**
> **PREPARATION TIME:** 5 minutes **COOKING TIME:** 20 minutes
> (mostly unattended)

This has been a long-time favorite of mine, and it's so easy to prepare and almost fat-free. I'm happy to include it here.

4 chicken breast fillets (about 1 lb)
⅓ cup honey
2 tablespoons brown mustard
4 cloves garlic, crushed

❧ PREHEAT oven to 350°F.

❧ SPRAY or brush an overproof dish with a little oil. Place chicken fillets in a single layer.

❧ MIX honey, mustard, and garlic together. Spread half of mixture over top of chicken fillets. Cover with aluminum foil.

❧ BAKE chicken in oven for 10 minutes. Uncover, turn chicken, and coat other side with rest of honey-mustard mixture. Bake, covered, for an additional 10 minutes, or until tender.

❧ SERVE with steamed or microwaved snow peas, corn, and baked potatoes.

Nutrients per serving
Fat: 2.9 g, Saturated fat: 0.7 g, Fiber: 0.5 g, Sodium: 208 g, Calories: 221

Tandoori Chicken Drumsticks

SERVES 4
PREPARATION TIME: 5 minutes (plus 1 hour marinating)
COOKING TIME: 20 minutes

This recipe is a favorite of Karen Kingham, a dietitian and colleague of mine who enjoys good food and loves to check out farmers' markets. It uses a commercial bottled paste, which saves time and yet gives an excellent flavor without the work!

4 tablespoons low-fat yogurt
4 tablespoons tandoori paste
8 chicken drumsticks, skin removed
chopped fresh cilantro, to garnish
4 poppadums (Indian flatbread)

Sauce
1 cup low-fat yogurt
1 small cucumber, peeled and diced
2 tablespoons chopped fresh cilantro

❥ COMBINE yogurt and tandoori paste in a small bowl to make a marinade.
❥ SCORE drumsticks diagonally with a sharp knife. Arrange in a shallow dish. Coat well with prepared marinade. Allow to marinate for at least 1 hour (or overnight in the refrigerator).
❥ REMOVE drumsticks from marinade, and grill for 20 minutes, or until fully cooked, turning during cooking.
❥ COMBINE sauce ingredients in a small bowl.
❥ COOK poppadums (follow packet directions).
❥ SERVE chicken on steamed basmati rice topped with sauce and cilantro. Accompany with a poppadum.

Nutrients per serving
Fat: 7.5 g, Saturated fat: 2.1 g, Fiber: 0.3 g, Sodium: 979 g, Calories: 243

Warm Chicken Salad with Orange and Walnuts

> **SERVES 6**
> **PREPARATION TIME:** 15 minutes **COOKING TIME:** 5 minutes

I love warm salads, and this one regularly appears in our house. The combination of orange, ginger, and walnuts with the lettuce and chicken is delicious. Lots of heart protectors here!

6 cups mixed lettuce leaves (mesclun)
12 oz snow peas, trimmed and halved
1 orange, peeled and segmented
½ cup sliced water chestnuts (or use 2 ribs celery, sliced)
2 chicken breast fillets (about ½ lb)
1 tablespoon canola oil
1 teaspoon grated fresh ginger
freshly ground black pepper
2 tablespoons chopped walnuts

Dressing
¼ cup orange juice
1 tablespoon walnut or canola oil
2 teaspoons grated orange rind
1 teaspoon Dijon mustard
1 teaspoon chopped fresh chives

- TEAR lettuce leaves into fork-size pieces, removing any brown edges. Toss in a salad bowl with snow peas. Add orange segments and water chestnuts.
- SLICE chicken finely into strips. Heat oil in a wok or deep frying pan. Stir-fry chicken strips and ginger for 3–4 minutes, until golden. Sprinkle with lots of pepper, and add to salad.
- PLACE dressing ingredients in a small screwtop jar, and shake well until blended.
- POUR dressing over salad. Toss to combine. Sprinkle with walnuts.

VARIATIONS
- Substitute 1 pork fillet (about 7 oz) for the chicken.
- Replace orange segments, juice, and rind, with finely sliced soft dried apricots. Use the same orange dressing.
- If you have leftover cooked chicken, substitute 3 cups diced chicken for the breasts, and warm in microwave before mixing with salad.

Nutrients per serving
Fat: 10.4 g, Saturated fat: 0.9 g, Fiber: 4.0 g, Sodium: 49 mg, Calories: 175,
Good for: folate, antioxidants

Vietnamese Chicken Salad with Mint and Cilantro

SERVES 4
PREPARATION TIME: 20 minutes **COOKING TIME:** 10 minutes

With its lightness and ultra-fresh ingredients, Vietnamese cuisine is starting to appear on health-conscious menus everywhere. Try this easy recipe, and you'll see why. It can be served cold or as a warm salad.

1 tablespoon peanut oil
2 skinless chicken thigh or breast fillets
(about 10 oz)
2 teaspoons fresh grated ginger
3 cups mixed lettuce leaves
1 bunch cilantro, stems removed
1 cup mint leaves
1 small red bell pepper, seeds removed
and sliced
6 shallots, sliced
7 oz snow peas, trimmed
12 cherry tomatoes, halved

Peanut dressing
⅓ cup crushed peanuts
2 tablespoons peanut oil
2 tablespoons lemon juice
1 tablespoon sugar
1 tablespoon fish sauce
1–2 chili peppers, seeded and sliced

➔ HEAT oil in a frying pan. Cook chicken for 5 minutes on both sides, until golden and cooked through. Smear ginger over each breast during cooking.
➔ REMOVE from pan. Slice thinly, and let cool.
➔ TOSS lettuce, cilantro, mint, pepper, shallots, peas, and tomatoes together with chicken in a serving bowl.

❥ PLACE all dressing ingredients in a small screwtop jar. Shake until sugar has dissolved. Pour over salad, and serve immediately.

VARIATION
- Substitute 3 cups diced leftover cooked chicken for the breasts or thighs, and warm in microwave before mixing with salad.

TIP
- Don't make dressing until just before serving or peanuts will turn soggy.

Nutrients per serving
Fat: 22.6 g, Saturated fat: 3.9 g, Fiber: 5.7 g, Sodium: 445 mg, Calories: 265, Good for: folate, antioxidants, nuts`

Easy Teriyaki Garlic Chicken

SERVES 4
PREPARATION TIME: 10 minutes **COOKING TIME:** 7 minutes

Quick and easy for when there's no time to cook!

1 tablespoon peanut oil
2 cloves garlic, crushed
1 teaspoon chopped chili pepper
1 teaspoon grated fresh ginger
2 tablespoons teriyaki sauce
4 chicken breasts, skin removed (about 1½ lb)
chopped fresh cilantro, to garnish
2 tablespoons chopped shallots, to garnish

Dressing
¼ cup orange juice
1 tablespoon walnut or canola oil
2 teaspoons grated orange rind
1 teaspoon Dijon mustard
1 teaspoon chopped fresh chives

❯ HEAT oil in pan. Add garlic, pepper, and ginger. Cook, stirring, for 1 minute until combined and heated through. Stir in teriyaki.
❯ PLACE chicken in pan, turning once to coat each piece evenly.
❯ REDUCE heat. Cook, covered, for 5–7 minutes, or until cooked through.
❯ SERVE with steamed noodles and pan-tossed Asian greens such as bok choy or gai lum. Garnish with cilantro and shallots.

Nutrients per serving
Fat: 7.5 g, Saturated fat: 1.5 g, Fiber: 0.3 g, Sodium: 129 mg, Calories: 176

❥ Five Ways to Enjoy Pasta and Rice ❥

Rice with Spinach and Pine Nuts

SERVES 4
PREPARATION TIME: 8 minutes **COOKING TIME:** 30 minutes
(mostly unattended)

With a green leaf salad, this easy rice dish can be a complete meatless meal, or it can double as a side dish to chicken or pork. It's a little like a risotto without all the stirring.

1 cup brown rice
1 onion, finely chopped
2 cups chicken stock or water
5–6 leaves fresh spinach
¼ cup grated low-fat Cheddar cheese
freshly ground black pepper
2 tablespoons pine nuts, toasted (see Tip, page 126)

❥ COMBINE rice, onion, and stock in a frying pan. Bring to a boil while stirring. Lower heat, cover, and simmer for 25 minutes.
❥ TRIM stalks from spinach, and shred finely. Add spinach to rice. Cook for 5 minutes, or until rice is tender and all the liquid absorbed.
❥ STIR in cheese.
❥ SERVE topped with pepper and pine nuts.

VARIATION
Instead of fresh spinach, you can use ½ cup frozen spinach (drain well first), 1 cup finely chopped celery, or ½ cup finely chopped fresh parsley or basil.

Nutrients per serving
Fat: 7.6 g, Saturated fat: 1.6 g, Fiber: 2.9 g, Sodium: 662 mg, Calories: 264, Good for: folate, whole grains

Quick Chicken and Mushroom Risotto

SERVES 4
PREPARATION TIME: 10 minutes **COOKING TIME:** 20 minutes

This super meal-in-one gives you carbohydrates, vegetables, and protein all together. It's a dish you can make ahead and reheat for lunch the next day.

2 tablespoons olive oil
1½ cups short-grain rice
1 chicken breast fillet, sliced into fine strips
4.5 oz mushrooms, sliced
1 cup fresh or frozen peas
½ red bell pepper, finely sliced
1 onion, chopped
1 cup chicken stock or water
½ cup tomato sauce
½ cup white wine
2 tablespoons chopped parsley
1 bay leaf
fresh basil leaves, to garnish

➤ HEAT oil in a large nonstick pan.
➤ ADD rice, chicken strips, mushrooms, peas, pepper, and onion. Cook for 2–3 minutes, stirring, until all ingredients are well coated in oil.
➤ ADD stock, sauce, wine, parsley, and bay leaf. Cover, and simmer, stirring occasionally to prevent sticking. Cook for 10–12 minutes, until all liquid is absorbed and rice is cooked through.
➤ REMOVE from heat, and let stand, covered, for 5 minutes. Remove bay leaf.
➤ SERVE garnished with basil and accompanied by a mixed leaf salad.

TIP
- You can use traditional Italian arborio rice to make this risotto, but cooking time will increase to about 30 minutes.

Nutrients per serving
Fat: 11.2 g, Saturated fat: 1.6 g, Fiber: 4.2 g, Sodium: 660 mg, Calories: 432, Good for: folate

Italian Sardine Pasta with Caper and Lemon Dressing

> **SERVES 4**
> **PREPARATION TIME:** 15 minutes **COOKING TIME:** 12 minutes

Sardines are an oily fish high in omega-3s. Easy and convenient in cans, most people just eat them as a snack. This is a tangy recipe that uses them in a different way.

12 oz fusilli or elbow pasta
1 bunch fresh asparagus, trimmed
and cut into pieces
1 bunch arugula, stalks trimmed
2 3-oz cans sardines in water,
drained and cut into large chunks
½ cup cherry tomatoes, halved
4 black olives
2 tablespoons shaved Parmesan cheese

Caper and lemon dressing

¼ cup extra virgin lemon dressing
¼ cup capers, drained and chopped
¼ cup chopped Italian parsley
juice of 1 lemon
1 teaspoon grated lemon rind
½ teaspoon cracked pepper

> ❥ BRING a large pot of water to a boil. Add the pasta, and stir well to prevent sticking. Reduce heat, and cook for 8–10 minutes, or until just tender. Drain pasta, then place in a large mixing bowl.
> ❥ MIX all dressing ingredients. Pour over pasta, tossing to combine.
> ❥ COOK asparagus in a saucepan of boiling water for 1–2 minutes, or until it has turned bright green (do not overcook—should be still crisp). Drain, and refresh under cold water.
> ❥ ADD asparagus to pasta, along with arugula, sardines, tomatoes, and olives. Toss well to combine.
> ❥ SERVE garnished with Parmesan cheese.

TIP

• This dish is a little higher in salt, but there are ways to minimize the salt if you need to. Use only half the olives (and slice them rather than serving whole), rinse the capers under cold water to remove their saltiness, and omit the Parmesan.

Nutrients per serving

Fat: 22.7 g, Saturated fat: 4.5 g, Fiber: 6.8 g, Sodium: 317 mg, Calories: 563, Good for: omega-3s, folate, low GI

Chicken and Pesto Pasta

SERVES 4
PREPARATION TIME: 10 minutes **COOKING TIME:** 10 minutes

These days, you can prepare meals so much faster thanks to the bottled and ready-made sauces now available, like the pesto used here. Many food companies have worked hard to cut out unnecessary fats, use fresh ingredients, and gradually reduce salt content.

8 oz linguini or fettuccini
1 tablespoon olive oil
½ barbecued chicken, skin removed
½ cup prepared pesto sauce
½ red bell pepper, seeds removed and sliced
4 shallots, sliced
2 oz bocconcini (fresh mozzarella nuggets), sliced
1 tablespoon sliced sun-dried tomatoes

- BRING a large pot of water to a boil. Add pasta, and stir well to prevent sticking. Reduce heat, and cook for 8–10 minutes, or until just tender. Drain, and toss with olive oil. Keep warm.
- BREAK chicken into pieces, discarding bones.
- TOSS chicken in hot pasta with pesto, pepper, and shallots over medium heat.
- SERVE topped with bocconcini and sun-dried tomatoes. Accompany with a mixed leaf salad and a seeded loaf of bread.

VARIATION
- Substitute 2 4-oz blocks firm tofu for the chicken, and skip the bocconcini.

TIP
- Use the chicken bones to make a delicious chicken stock. Simply bring to a boil with onion, carrot, celery, peppercorns, and a few favorite herbs. Use as the basis for soup or in casseroles. Freeze until needed.

Nutrients per serving
Fat: 31.0 g, Saturated fat: 3.8 g, Fiber: 3.4 g, Sodium: 871 mg, Calories: 602,
Good for: folate, antioxidants, low GI

Salmon Vegetable Macaroni Toss

> **SERVES 4**
> **PREPARATION TIME:** 10 minutes **COOKING TIME:** 18 minutes

This is a delightfully simple way to make use of a can of salmon—my idea of a lazy Sunday night dinner.

1 lb macaroni (elbows, spirals, or other small pasta)
1 tablespoon olive oil
2 cups diced vegetables (mixture of 2 or 3 kinds—zucchini, mushroom, red bell pepper, celery, snow peas, cooked green peas, corn)
1 onion, finely chopped
1 teaspoon crushed garlic
3 chopped ripe tomatoes or 1 cup tomato sauce
7-oz can pink or red salmon, flaked
chopped fresh basil or parsley

❯ BRING a large pot of water to a boil. Add pasta, and stir well to prevent sticking. Reduce heat. Cook for 8–10 minutes, or until just tender.

❯ DRAIN well, and place in a large pasta bowl for serving. Keep warm while preparing sauce.

❯ HEAT oil in a nonstick pan, and sauté vegetables, onion, and garlic for 3–4 minutes. Add tomatoes (plus a little water if necessary). Cook, covered, over gentle heat for another 3 minutes, stirring once or twice.

❯ ADD salmon to sauce along with any liquid from the can. Spoon sauce over macaroni, tossing well to combine.

❯ SERVE topped with basil.

Nutrients per serving
Fat 10.2 g, Saturated fat 2.0 g, Fiber 8.2 g, Sodium 254 mg, Calories 557,
Good for: omega-3, folate, antioxidants, low GI

❧ Five Vegetarian Dishes ❧

Stir-fry of Tofu, Asparagus, and Asian Greens

SERVES 4
PREPARATION TIME: 15 minutes **COOKING TIME:** 7 minutes

Stir-fries are an easy way to incorporate more tofu into your diet. The tofu, being bland in taste, takes on the flavors of the other ingredients.

10 oz firm tofu, sliced
2 tablespoons reduced-sodium soy sauce
1 tablespoon peanut or canola oil
1 teaspoon grated fresh ginger
1 clove garlic, crushed
1 bunch asparagus, trimmed and halved
3 oz snow peas, trimmed
3 oz baby corn, halved lengthwise (or 15-oz can, drained)
4 cups mixed Asian greens, chopped (see Note)
4 oz mushrooms, sliced
1 tablespoon oyster sauce
1 tablespoon dry sherry
½ cup bamboo shoots

❧ PLACE tofu and soy sauce in a bowl. Marinate for 5 minutes. Heat oil in a wok, and stir-fry tofu until golden. Drain on paper towel, and set aside.

❧ ADD ginger and garlic to the wok. Stir-fry for 30 seconds. Add asparagus, snow peas, and baby corn. Toss to combine, and stir-fry for 1–2 minutes.

❧ ADD Asian greens and mushrooms to wok, along with tofu, oyster sauce, and sherry. Stir-fry for 2 minutes, or until heated through. Add bamboo shoots.

❧ SERVE with rice or noodles.

NOTE
- Asian greens include bok choy (also called buck or pak choy), baby bok choy, choy sum (Chinese flowering cabbage), gai lum (Chinese broccoli), and wong bok (Chinese cabbage). Any of these can be used in this recipe—simply remove any yellowed or wilted outer leaves, and chop roughly. If not available in your area, alternatives are baby spinach leaves or shredded cabbage.

Nutrients per serving
Fat: 17.4 g, Saturated fat: 1.3 g, Fiber: 6.6 g, Sodium: 699 mg, Calories: 202,
Good for: folate, antioxidants, soy protein

Barbecued Rosemary Vegetable Kebabs

SERVES 4
PREPARATION TIME: 10 minutes **COOKING TIME:** 20 minutes

Vegetarian? These kebabs are perfect to throw on the barbecue when all the carnivores are cooking their steaks. I bet the carnivores will want some too!

4 small potatoes, halved
1 onion, halved and separated
2 zucchini, cut into thick slices
8 mushrooms
1 red bell pepper, seeds removed
and quartered
4 small yellow squash
8 cherry tomatoes
16 fresh rosemary sprigs, about 1" long
8 bamboo skewers, soaked
oil spray

Tzatziki dipping sauce
1 cup plain low-fat yogurt
1 small cucumber, peeled and finely chopped
2–3 cloves garlic, crushed
1 tablespoon fresh chopped mint
squeeze of lemon juice
freshly ground black pepper

❯ PARBOIL potatoes for 5 minutes. Cool.
❯ THREAD vegetables and rosemary sprigs onto skewers, and spray with oil.
❯ BARBECUE or cook under a preheated broiler for 10 minutes, spraying if needed with extra oil. Turn frequently during cooking.
❯ PREPARE dipping sauce by combining all ingredients. Serve with vegetable kebabs.

TIP
- Soak bamboo skewers in water for 15–30 minutes before using, to prevent them from burning.

VARIATIONS
- In place of rosemary, substitute individual garlic cloves threaded on the skewers between the vegetables.
- Small pieces of fresh chopped chili pepper threaded onto each skewer are nice if you like hot food.

Nutrients per serving
Fat: 1.2 g, Saturated fat: 0.2 g, Fiber: 5.4 g, Sodium: 62 mg, Calories: 119,
Good for: folate

Mediterranean pasta

SERVES 4
PREPARATION TIME: 15 minutes **COOKING TIME:** 15 minutes

Tomatoes have made headlines for their rich content of lycopene, a powerful antioxidant that gives them their red color. During cooking, the lycopene is released from within the cells, so it's better absorbed from cooked and pureed tomatoes than from fresh.

12 oz spaghetti or pasta of your choice
¼ cup olive oil
1 onion, chopped
2 cloves garlic, crushed
7–8 very ripe tomatoes, chopped
¼ cup pitted black olives
1 teaspoon grated lemon rind
2 tablespoons chopped basil

❯ COOK spaghetti in a large saucepan of boiling water over medium heat for 10 minutes, or until al dente. Drain well. Place in a large serving bowl. Keep warm.
❯ HEAT oil in a frying pan. Sauté onion and garlic until tender.
❯ ADD tomatoes, olives, rind and basil. Simmer, covered, for 10–15 minutes, or until tomatoes are soft and a sauce consistency is achieved.
❯ TOSS with hot pasta. Serve with crusty bread and a mixed leaf salad.

Nutrients per serving
Fat: 16.7 g, Saturated fat: 2.4 g, Fiber: 8.9 g, Sodium: 23 mg, Calories: 499,
Good for: folate, antioxidants, low GI

Potato, Chickpea, and Cashew Curry

> **SERVES 6**
> **PREPARATION TIME:** 15 minutes **COOKING TIME:** 40 minutes
> (mostly unattended)

This is a wonderful vegetarian recipe from Sally James, talented Australian chef and author. Sally's creative recipes reflect her love of food and her background at Australia's Heart Foundation and the Victor Chang Cardiac Research Institute. This dish tastes as good as it sounds!

1 tablespoon olive oil
1 teaspoon mustard seeds
1 teaspoon coriander seeds
1 teaspoon cumin seeds
1 tablespoon fresh grated ginger
1 large onion, chopped
1 tablespoon curry paste (mild or hot to taste)
2 medium potatoes
13 oz cooked or canned chickpeas
13-oz can diced tomatoes, no added salt
½ cup vegetable stock or water
½ cup cashews, toasted (see Tip, page 126)

♦ HEAT oil in a large, heavy saucepan. Cook the mustard, coriander, and cumin seeds until they start to pop.
♦ ADD the ginger, onion, and curry paste. Cook for 2–3 minutes, or until onion is soft.
♦ ADD the potatoes, chickpeas, tomatoes, and stock, and bring to a boil. Reduce heat. Simmer, covered, for 20–30 minutes, or until potatoes are tender, adding more water if necessary.
♦ STIR in cashews, and serve with steamed green beans.

Nutrients per serving
Fat: 11.9 g, Saturated fat: n/a, Fiber: 5.4 g, Sodium: 374 mg, Calories: 229,
Good for: soluble fiber, folate, antioxidants, nuts

❧ Things to Do with Bread ❧

Spicy Soy Burgers with
Yogurt Chutney Dressing

> **SERVES 4**
> **PREPARATION TIME:** 30 minutes **COOKING TIME:** 10 minutes

Everyone loves a burger, and if you're vegetarian, there's no reason to miss out with these yummy soybean versions. Any bean can be used—soaked and boiled or canned—and lentils work well too.

1 cup cooked soybeans (or 1 10-oz can soybeans)
1 onion, grated
3 cloves garlic, crushed
1 medium carrot, grated
1 cup soft whole grain bread crumbs
2 tablespoons wheat germ + 2 additional teaspoons
1 egg, beaten
2 tablespoons curry paste or 2 teaspoons curry powder
2 tablespoons chopped fresh parsley
2 teaspoons grated fresh ginger
2 tablespoons sesame seeds
2 tablespoons peanut oil
8 whole grain rolls, muffins, or pitas
8 leaves lettuce
2 tomatoes, sliced

Yogurt sauce
1 cup plain low-fat yogurt
½ cup mango chutney
1 tablespoon chopped fresh cilantro

❧ DRAIN and rinse canned beans, if using, to remove jellied liquid. Blend beans in a food processor until pureed but not too smooth. Mix in onion, garlic, carrot, bread crumbs, wheat germ, egg, curry paste, parsley, and ginger. Form into 8 patties. Roll in combined sesame seeds and extra wheat germ until coated evenly. Heat oil in a large nonstick pan. Add burgers. Cook for about 5 minutes on each side, until golden brown. Alternatively, bake at 350°F for 30 minutes, turning once.

❥ COMBINE all sauce ingredients.

❥ SERVE burgers hot on toasted rolls with lettuce, tomato, and yogurt sauce.

Nutrients per serving
Fat: 19.9 g, Saturated fat: 3.6 g, Fiber: 15.7 g, Sodium: 1,272 mg, Calories: 562, Good for: soluble fiber, folate, soy protein, low GI

Homemade Pizza with Artichoke and Roasted Red Bell Pepper

SERVES 4
PREPARATION TIME: 10 minutes **COOKING TIME:** 15 minutes

Pizza pleases almost everyone! By choosing the right toppings, you can make it healthy and lower in fat.

> 2 12" pizza bases or 4 whole grain pitas
> 1 cup thick tomato sauce or 1 cup pesto
> 6 artichoke hearts, drained and sliced
> 1 7-oz can tuna in springwater, drained
> 12 strips roasted red bell pepper
> 1 cup mushrooms, sliced
> 4 bocconcini (fresh mozzarella nuggets), about 2 oz each, sliced or
> 2 cups grated reduced-fat mozzarella cheese
> fresh basil leaves or Italian parsley

➤ PREHEAT oven to 400°F.
➤ SPRAY or brush a baking tray with oil. Place base on the prepared tray. (If you prefer your pizza crisp and crunchy, simply place the assembled pizza directly on the oven rack.)
➤ SPREAD tomato sauce over the base (or over split, lightly toasted pitas).
➤ ARRANGE artichokes, tuna, pepper, mushrooms, and slices of bocconcini on top.
➤ BAKE for 8–10 minutes, or until cheese melts a little and just browns. Top with basil leaves. Serve with a mixed leaf salad.

VARIATIONS
• Substitute thinly sliced zucchini or fennel or some sliced sun-dried tomatoes in place of the pepper and mushrooms.
• In place of the tuna, try 2.5 oz smoked salmon slices, 3.5 oz scallops, marinara mix from your fish market, or ½ cup diced lean ham.

Nutrients per serving
Fat: 13.1 g, Saturated fat: 7.3 g, Fiber: 7.1 g, Sodium: 1,408 mg, Calories: 392, Good for: omega-3s, folate, whole grains

Open Sandwich of Ham and Sun-dried Tomato

SERVES 4
PREPARATION TIME: 8 minutes **COOKING TIME:** nil

Easy to assemble, this sandwich is designed to be eaten with a fork and knife (good for dieters, as this slows down your rate of eating). It makes a heartier lunch than just an ordinary sandwich. You can also serve it on toasted whole grain bread or muffins.

4 thick slices rye bread
6 tablespoons cottage cheese or low-fat mayonnaise
7 oz chipped ham
4 tablespoons spiced tomato relish (chutney)
½ cup sun-dried tomato halves
basil leaves

➤ PLACE each slice of bread on a serving plate. Spread with cottage cheese.
➤ ARRANGE ham over the cottage cheese, then top with relish, tomatoes, and basil.

VARIATIONS
• Baked ricotta (see page 193), thin slices of smoked salmon, rings of red Spanish onion, capers, lemon juice, and fresh dill
• Sliced avocado, thinly sliced rare roast beef, tomato slices, and arugula
• A dollop of cottage cheese, lettuce, canned drained sardines, and lemon wedges
• Mayonnaise, cooked chicken breast, chopped celery, walnut halves, and slices of red-skinned apple

Nutrients per serving
Fat: 5.4 g, Saturated fat: 1.5 g, Fiber: 4.8 g, Sodium: 1,354 mg, Calories: 250, Good for: low GI, whole grains

Tomato and Basil Bruscetta

SERVES 4
PREPARATION TIME: 10 minutes **COOKING TIME:** 5 minutes

Light and fresh, this makes an easy lunch or a great pre-dinner nibble. You can prepare the tomato ahead, then toast the bread and add the topping at the last minute.

12 thick rounds wood-fired bread
1 tablespoon extra-virgin olive oil
2 cloves garlic, crushed
5–6 large ripe plum tomatoes
2 shallots, finely sliced
¼ cup basil leaves, chopped
2 teaspoons balsamic vinegar
freshly ground black pepper

❥ PREHEAT broiler.
❥ TOAST bread lightly under broiler on both sides, until just golden (this can also be done in a wide toaster). Brush bread with oil, smear garlic over top.
❥ DICE tomatoes, removing central line of seeds if desired. Toss with shallots, basil, vinegar, and pepper.
❥ TOP each slice of bread with tomato mixture. Serve immediately.

VARIATION
• Bruscetta can also be grilled with a little cheese and served hot. Top with thinly sliced mozzarella or bocconcini. Grill for 2 minutes, or until heated through.

Nutrients per serving
Fat: 7.6 g, Saturated fat: 1.3 g, Fiber: 4.8 g, Sodium: 485 mg, Calories: 321, Good for: folate, antioxidants

Beef, Avocado, and Basil Melt

SERVES 4
PREPARATION TIME: 10 minutes **COOKING TIME:** 5 minutes

Use this recipe as a "template" for your own favorite toppings. For anyone who misses the taste of salt, try to include strongly aromatic ingredients like the fresh basil in this recipe, and you won't notice the lack of salt.

8 slices whole grain bread
1 avocado, peeled and sliced
8 thin slices roast beef or lamb
2–3 tomatoes, sliced thickly
⅓ cup chopped fresh basil
8 slices reduced-fat mozzarella cheese
freshly ground black pepper

❥ TOAST bread lightly, on one side only, under a preheated broiler. Spread untoasted side with avocado. Arrange beef, tomatoes, and basil on avocado. Top with cheese. Season with black pepper.

❥ PLACE under broiler again, and cook for 2–3 minutes, or until heated and cheese is melted.

VARIATION
• Substitute whatever you have in the kitchen: fresh red bell pepper, sun-dried tomatoes, marinated eggplant, sliced artichoke hearts, smoked chicken, canned salmon or tuna.

Nutrients per serving
Fat: 28.5 g, Saturated fat: 9.2 g, Fiber: 7.0 g, Sodium: 555 mg, Calories: 507, Good for: folate

Lavash Toast with Cumin Seed

SERVES 12
PREPARATION TIME: 10 minutes **COOKING TIME:** 5 minutes

Instead of high-fat chips and crackers, serve these crunchy toast triangles with dips, or munch on them as a snack. They keep well for 2–3 weeks.

> 4 pieces lavash bread (around 3 oz)
> 2 tablespoons olive oil, for brushing (or use oil spray)
> 1 tablespoon cumin seed

- PREHEAT oven to 350°F.
- BRUSH or spray one side of each lavash bread lightly with oil.
- CUT each into triangles, and sprinkle with seeds.
- PLACE oiled side up, in a single layer, on baking trays lined with wax paper.
- BAKE in oven for 4–5 minutes, or until just golden. Store in airtight containers.

VARIATION
- In place of cumin, substitute lemon pepper, cracked pepper, sesame seeds, poppy seeds, or linseeds.

Nutrients per serving
Fat: 3.4 g, Saturated fat: 0.5 g, Fiber: 0.3 g, Sodium: 42 mg, Calories: 52

❧ Five Super Salads ❧

Fruit and Nut Coleslaw

> **SERVES 4–6**
> **PREPARATION TIME:** 20 minutes **COOKING TIME:** nil

An unusual variation on the standard coleslaw theme.

2 cups finely shredded red cabbage
2 cups finely shredded green cabbage
1 carrot, grated
1 green apple, finely diced
4 shallots, sliced
½ cup sliced dried apricots
¼ cup slivered almonds
½ cup low-fat coleslaw dressing

❧ COMBINE cabbages, carrot, apple, shallots, apricots, and almonds in a large bowl.
❧ MIX in coleslaw dressing, tossing to coat all ingredients.
❧ CHILL before serving.

Nutrients per serving
Fat: 4.4 g, Saturated fat: 0.3 g, Fiber: 4.9 g, Sodium: 176 mg, Calories: 112,
Good for: folate, antioxidants

Salad of Roasted Vegetables with Baked Ricotta and Arugula

SERVES 4
PREPARATION TIME: 30 minutes **COOKING TIME:** 25 minutes

A good salad for cooler days or when you're tired of lettuce and cucumber. Any vegetables that can be char-grilled can be used.

¼ quantity Baked Ricotta (page 193) or 8 oz baked ricotta from a
   good delicatessen
1 red bell pepper
3 zucchini, sliced lengthwise
4 baby eggplants, halved lengthwise
1 bunch asparagus, trimmed
6 plum tomatoes, halved lengthwise
1 bunch arugula
2 tablespoons Parmesan cheese shavings

Dressing
2 tablespoons extra-virgin olive oil
2 teaspoons balsamic vinegar
freshly ground black pepper

✦ MAKE Baked Ricotta with chopped herbs, lemon rind, and pepper as suggested in the Variation (page 193). Cool, and slice half of it (or all of bought ricotta) into small wedges or strips.
✦ PLACE bell pepper under a preheated hot broiler. Cook 3–4 minutes on each side, until pepper is charred. Place in a bowl. Cover with plastic wrap. When cool, peel away blackened skin. Cut in half, and remove seeds and membranes. Cut into thick slices. Set aside.
✦ BRUSH preheated broiler with a little oil. Cook zucchini, eggplant, asparagus, and tomatoes for 3–5 minutes each side, until golden and tender.
✦ PLACE in a bowl with torn arugula leaves and bell pepper.
✦ COMBINE ingredients for dressing in a screwtop jar, and shake well

❥ DRIZZLE vegetables with dressing. Serve topped with wedges of ricotta and Parmesan.

Nutrients per serving
Fat: 18.7 g, Saturated fat: 6.9 g, Fiber: 4.9 g, Sodium: 211 mg, Calories: 243, Good for: folate, antioxidants, low GI

Thai Beef Salad

SERVES 4
PREPARATION TIME: 15 minutes **COOKING TIME:** 10 minutes

A substantial salad rich with the fragrance of cilantro, lime, chili pepper, onion, and mint. Also works well with cold lamb or pork.

1 lb lean beef (fillet or rump)
1 red bell pepper, seeds removed and sliced
1 red onion, finely sliced
2 tablespoons chopped mint
4 cups mixed lettuce leaves (mesclun)
8 oz cherry tomatoes, halved
1–2 red chili peppers, sliced finely (or more to taste)
cilantro sprigs

Dressing
⅓ cup lime or lemon juice
2 cloves garlic, crushed
freshly ground black pepper
2 teaspoons fish sauce
1 teaspoon sugar

♦ COOK beef on a hot grill or under a broiler for 5 minutes each side. In this recipe, steak is best rare. Let stand for 5 minutes.
♦ SLICE beef into thin pieces or strips. Toss in a bowl with red bell pepper, onion, and mint.
♦ COMBINE ingredients for dressing in a screwtop jar, and shake well. Pour dressing over meat mixture.
♦ ARRANGE lettuce leaves on a large platter.
   Top with the beef mixture, and scatter with tomato halves.
♦ GARNISH with chili peppers and cilantro. Serve with whole grain bread.

Nutrients per serving
Fat: 4.4 g, Saturated fat: 1.8 g, Fiber: 2.3 g, Sodium: 188 mg, Calories: 152, Good for: folate, antioxidants, low GI

Salmon, Baby Spinach, and Couscous Salad

> **SERVES 4**
> **PREPARATION TIME:** 10 minutes **COOKING TIME:** 3 minutes

Lots of heart protectors in this quick and easy salad, including lemon, fish, tomatoes, parsley, onions, spinach, and nuts.

1¼ cups (10 oz) vegetable stock or water
1 cup (7 oz) couscous
1 tablespoon lemon juice
1 tablespoon extra-virgin olive oil
1 teaspoon grated lemon rind
7-oz can pink or red salmon, drained
8 cherry tomatoes, halved
½ cup chopped Italian parsley
2–3 shallots, finely chopped
freshly ground black pepper
2 cups baby spinach leaves
¼ cup pine nuts, toasted (see Tip, page 126)

❧ BOIL stock in a medium-size stock pot. Remove from heat. Stir in couscous. Cover, and let swell for 2 minutes. Stir again with a fork to separate the grains.
❧ SPOON into a shallow bowl. Fluff with a fork to separate. Place in the refrigerator to cool for 5 minutes. Add juice, oil, and rind.
❧ FLAKE salmon, and place in a salad bowl with tomatoes, parsley, shallots (green and white stems), and pepper. Spoon couscous mixture into bowl. Mix all ingredients well.
❧ SERVE on spinach leaves, topped with pine nuts.

TIP
• You will need ½ a lemon for the rind and juice for this recipe.

Nutrients per serving
Fat: 16.1 g, Saturated fat: 2.2 g, Fiber: 4.4 g, Sodium: 587 mg, Calories: 233,
Good for: omega-3s, folate, antioxidants, nuts, low G

Smoked Chicken Summer Salad with Apricot-Mustard Dressing

> **SERVES 4**
> **PREPARATION TIME:** 15 minutes **COOKING TIME:** nil

This is an unusual salad, with two fruit elements that counter-balance the chicken and avocado.

4 cups mixed lettuce leaves (mesclun)
1 smoked chicken, bones removed, sliced
½ avocado, sliced
½ cup sliced sun-dried tomatoes
½ cup seedless white grapes
½ cup pine nuts, toasted (see Tip, page 126)

Apricot-mustard dressing
½ cup apricot nectar
2 tablespoons canola oil
1 tablespoon red wine vinegar
1–2 teaspoons brown mustard

🌢 ARRANGE lettuce, chicken, avocado, tomatoes, grapes, and nuts on a serving platter.
🌢 COMBINE all dressing ingredients in a jar, and shake well to mix.
🌢 POUR dressing over salad just prior to serving.

Nutrients per serving
Fat: 32.8 g, Saturated fat: 5.1 g, Fiber: 3.1 g, Sodium: 158 mg, Calories: 698,
Good for: folate, antioxidants, nuts, low GI

❥ Five Ways to End a Meal ❥

Ricotta with Baked Nectarines

> **SERVES 4**
> **PREPARATION TIME:** 10 minutes **COOKING TIME:** 5 minutes

When stone fruit are in season, try this stunning and easy dessert—everyone loves it! It can't be done until the last minute, but it's very quick. Make sure you buy soft fresh ricotta from a deli, not the type in a carton from the supermarket.

4 ripe nectarines
4 tablespoons brown sugar
8 oz fresh ricotta
2 tablespoons honey

❥ CUT nectarines into halves, and remove stones. Place cut side up on a baking tray that has been lined with wax paper.

❥ TOP each nectarine half with a ½ tablespoon sugar, spreading it over the sides and into the central well with a teaspoon.

❥ PLACE under a hot broiler for 5 minutes, or until sugar has melted and nectarines are just golden.

❥ SPOON 3–4 tablespoons of ricotta onto each of four dessert plates. Drizzle honey on top. Arrange two nectarine halves on each plate.

VARIATIONS
• Peaches or apricots can replace the nectarines, depending on what's in season.
• Substitute canned peach halves or apricots if fresh ones are out of season, but drain well on paper towels first, and reduce the cooking time.
• In place of ricotta, serve with a scoop of reduced-fat vanilla ice cream.

Nutrients per serving
Fat: 7.1 g, Saturated fat: 4.5 g, Fiber: 1.8 g, Sodium: 130 mg, Calories: 221, Good for: low GI

Lisa Yates' Low-fat Pavlova

SERVES 8
PREPARATION TIME: 20 minutes **COOKING TIME:**3 hours
(unattended)

Dietitian Lisa Yates has given me her favorite dessert recipe that, apart from being a national icon, makes a stunning finish to a meal. You'll think it's indulgent but Lisa's cleverly substituted low-fat yogurt for the cream, and the meringue has almost no fat.

6 egg whites at room temperature
pinch of cream of tartar
2 cups sugar
1 tablespoon cornstarch, sifted
2 teaspoons white vinegar
1 teaspoon vanilla essence

Topping
1 8-oz carton low-fat vanilla yogurt
7 oz strawberries, sliced
3–4 kiwifruit, sliced
pulp of 3–4 passionfruit

- PREHEAT oven to 300°F. Cut a sheet of wax paper 10" square. Draw a circle of 9" diameter on the paper. Place it on a greased tray drawn side down.
- WHISK the egg whites and cream of tartar together in a clean dry bowl using an electric mixer for 3–4 minutes, or until soft peaks form.
- ADD the sugar a spoon at a time, whisking well after each addition until meringue is thick and glossy (takes about 10 minutes).
- ADD cornstarch, vinegar, and vanilla. Gently fold through using a spatula. Spread meringue onto the prepared tray using the circle as a guide.
- BAKE for 1 hour, or until crisp. Turn the oven off. Allow the meringue to cool in the oven for 1–2 hours with the door slightly open.

❯ SLIDE the meringue off the paper onto a serving plate. Spread with yogurt, and arrange sliced fruit on top. Drizzle with passion-fruit before serving.

VARIATION
- Use any fruit you prefer: sliced banana, raspberries, blueberries, white grapes, slices of peaches or nectarines, mango, and fresh pineapple are all good.

Nutrients per serving
Fat: 0.2 g, Saturated fat: 0.0 g, Fiber: 3.3 g, Sodium: 71 mg, Calories: 279

Fresh Plum and Ricotta Strudel

> **SERVES 6**
> **PREPARATION TIME:** 20 minutes **COOKING TIME:** 25 minutes
> (mostly unattended)

Plums and other blue-red fruit, such as cherries, blueberries, and cranberries, are rich in a particular type of antioxidant known as anthocyanin.

Here's a low-fat version of strudel using plums instead of apples.

    1½ tablespoons soft margarine
    ⅓ cup brown sugar
    ½ cup fresh whole grain bread crumbs (3 slices)
    ½ teaspoon cinnamon
    8 oz fresh plums (about 4) or 14 oz can plums, drained well
    6 sheets phyllo pastry
    4 oz ricotta

❧ PREHEAT oven to 375°F.
❧ MELT margarine in a saucepan. Add sugar (reserving 2 teaspoons). Cook over moderate heat for 1 minute, until mixture bubbles. Remove from heat. Add bread crumbs and cinnamon. Stir well to break up any lumps. Let cool.
❧ HALVE plums, remove stones, and slice thinly.
❧ LAY two sheets of phyllo pastry on top of one another, spraying the uppermost sheet with oil. Sprinkle with one-third of the crumb mixture, and top with two more sheets. Spray top sheet with oil, and add another third of the crumb mixture. Top with remaining two sheets, and sprinkle with final third of the crumbs.
❧ SPREAD ricotta along one edge of pastry. Arrange plums on top of ricotta. Sprinkle with reserved 2 teaspoons sugar. Roll up pastry lengthwise, similar to a Swiss roll.
❧ TRANSFER to a lightly oiled baking tray. Spray top with oil. Bake for 10 minutes. Reduce heat to 350°F and bake an additional 10 minutes, until crisp and brown.

❥ SERVE warm with low-fat vanilla ice cream.

Nutrients per serving
Fat: 6.9 g, Saturated fat: 2.9 g, Fiber: 2.9 g, Sodium: 232 mg, Calories: 204,
Good for: antioxidants, low GI

Winter Compote of Dried Fruit Infused with Orange, Tea, and Spices

---

SERVES 6
PREPARATION TIME: 5 minutes
(plus 4 hours marinating time) **COOKING TIME:** nil

If you love dried fruit, like me, you'll love this dessert. It's an old-fashioned recipe but has virtually no fat except what you add from the almonds and yogurt.

12 dried apricots
12 prunes, pitted
12 dried apple rings
12 dried peach halves
6 dried figs (optional)
3–4 cloves
1 cinnamon stick
curl of orange rind
1 cup warm black tea or water
1 orange, peeled and sliced
vanilla low-fat yogurt
¼ cup flaked almonds, toasted (see Tip, page 126)

❥ PLACE apricots, prunes, apple rings, peaches, figs, cloves, cinnamon, and rind in a large glass or ceramic bowl.
❥ ADD tea. Cover, and refrigerate overnight or for at least 4 hours.
❥ BEFORE serving, remove cloves, cinnamon, and rind from compote. Add orange slices.
❥ SERVE topped with yogurt and almonds.

Nutrients per serving
Fat: 3.1 g, Saturated fat: 0.2 g, Fiber: 8.1 g, Sodium: 28 mg, Calories: 192,
Good for: soluble fiber, antioxidants, low GI

Persian Oranges
with Wine and Cloves

SERVES 4
PREPARATION TIME: 10 minutes
(plus 1-2 hours marinating time) **COOKING TIME:** 5 minutes

A refreshing tangy dessert that makes use of the wonderful navel oranges in season during winter. Perfect to serve after a curry or hot and spicy main course.

6 navel oranges
juice of 1 orange (about ½ cup)
½ cup white wine
¼ cup sugar
4–5 cloves

Yogurt topping
8-oz carton plain low-fat natural yogurt
2 tablespoons honey
grated rind of 1 orange
pinch of cinnamon

➤ PEEL oranges, and slice thinly. Arrange in a serving bowl.
➤ PLACE orange juice, wine, and sugar in a small saucepan, and heat gently to dissolve sugar. Pour over oranges, and add cloves.
➤ COVER, and marinate for 1–2 hours (can also be made the day before and refrigerated overnight).
➤ MIX yogurt topping ingredients in a small bowl until well combined.
➤ SERVE oranges with yogurt topping.

VARIATION
• Fresh pineapple, diced canteloupe, or sliced banana (or a mix of any of these) can also be used in place of the oranges.

Nutrients per serving
Fat: 0.4 g, Saturatred fat: 0.1 g, Fiber: 5.0 g, Sodium: 54 mg, Calories: 246, Good for: folate, antioxidants, low GI

❥ Five Sweet Treats ❥

Banana Bran Muffins

MAKES 12
PREPARATION TIME: 15 minutes **COOKING TIME:** 20 minutes
(unattended)

These low-fat muffins are quick and easy to bake and make a great snack or lunch box treat.

1 cup bran cereal
1 cup low-fat milk
1 egg, lightly beaten
2 tablespoons brown sugar
1 large ripe banana
2 tablespoons soft margarine
1 ¼ cups self-rising flour
¼ teaspoon cinnamon

❥ PREHEAT oven to 350°F.
❥ PLACE cereal in a mixing bowl. Add milk, egg, and sugar. Mix to combine. Let stand for 10 minutes.
❥ MASH banana with margarine. Stir into bran mixture. Add sifted flour and cinnamon. Mix with a wooden spoon until almost combined.
❥ SPOON into a 12-cup large muffin tray that has been sprayed or lightly oiled.
❥ BAKE for 20 minutes, or until golden brown.

VARIATION
• Add 2 tablespoons raisins with the flour.
• Sprinkle with flaked almonds before baking.

Nutrients per serving
Fat: 3.4 g, Saturated fat: 0.7 g, Fiber: 2.4 g, Sodium: 200 mg, Calories: 119,
Good for: folate

Kaye's Honey and Apple Muffins

> **MAKES 12**
> **PREPARATION TIME:** 30 minutes **COOKING TIME:** 20 minutes
> (unattended)

Andrew May, one of Australia's leading fitness experts and personal trainers, loves this recipe, which was given to him by Kaye Goldsmith from Hobart. After being stuck on the dieting roller coaster for years, Kay has totally changed the way she and her family eat, exercise, and enjoy life! She has also lost more than a foot from her waistline and is now a fitness leader (at the young age of 60).

¼ cup soft margarine
¼ cup honey
2 eggs (or 1 egg and 1 egg white)
½ teaspoon vanilla essence
1 cup low-fat plain yogurt
1 cup peeled diced apple
2 cups self-rising flour
½ teaspoon nutmeg

❥ PREHEAT oven to 400°F. Grease a large 12-cup muffin pan lightly with oil spray.
❥ BLEND margarine and honey. Beat in eggs and vanilla.
❥ ADD yogurt and apple. Gently fold in sifted flour and nutmeg.
❥ SPOON into prepared pan, and bake for 20 minutes. Cool in pan for 5–10 minutes.

Nutrients per serving
Fat: 5.1 g, Saturated fat: 1.1 g, Fiber: 1.1 g, Sodium: 230 mg, Calories: 188

Date and Almond Cake

> **MAKES 12**
> **PREPARATION TIME:** 30 minutes **COOKING TIME:** 30 minutes
> (unattended)

This easy cake is an update of a family favorite from food consultant Jennene Plummer. It's much lower in fat than a normal cake, and the dates and nuts add fiber and antioxidants.

3 oz soft margarine
1 cup brown sugar
1 egg
1½ cups self-rising flour
1 cup chopped dates
¼ cup slivered almonds

- ➤ PREHEAT oven to 350°F.
- ➤ CREAM margarine and sugar together. Add egg, and beat well.
- ➤ FOLD in sifted flour, followed by dates.
- ➤ SPRAY a 7" x 11" baking tin with oil spray.
- ➤ SPOON mixture into tin, smoothing top. Sprinkle almonds over.
- ➤ BAKE for 30 minutes, or until golden brown. Cool in tin, cut into squares, and store in airtight container.

TIP
- Chop dates with a pair of scissors, rather than a knife, to make the job easier.

Nutrients per serving
Fat: 7.3 g, Saturated fat: 2.2 g, Fiber: 1.9 g, Sodium: 164 mg, Calories: 25,
Good for: soluble fiber

My Favorite Carrot Cake

8 SLICES
PREPARATION TIME: 30 minutes **COOKING TIME:** 1 hour
(unattended)

I love a good carrot cake, and this one works well every time. It's a good example of how you can modify some of your favorite baking recipes to cut back on the fat or change the type of fat used. It keeps well for up to one week.

2 cups grated carrot (2 medium carrots)
¼ cup pecans or walnuts, chopped
½ cup raisins
¾ cup canola oil or light olive oil
1 cup brown sugar, lightly packed
2 teaspoons cinnamon
3 eggs
1½ cups whole grain self-rising flour
1 teaspoon bicarbonate of soda

- PREHEAT oven to 350°F. Line a 4" x 8" loaf pan with wax paper.
- PLACE carrots, pecans, and raisins in a large mixing bowl. Set aside. BEAT oil until light and frothy in another bowl. Add sugar and cinnamon. Beat until smooth. Add eggs, one at a time, and continue beating until thick.
- FOLD in sifted flour and soda. Add flour mixture to prepared carrot mixture. Mix well.
- SPOON into prepared loaf pan and smooth top. Bake for 1 hour, or until done when tested. Let cool in pan for 5 minutes before turning out to cool on a wire rack.

Nutrients per serving
Fat: 27.7 g, Saturated fat: 2.4 g, Fiber: 4.7 g, Sodium: 286 mg, Calories: 439,
Good for: antioxidants

Apricot Oat Munchies

MAKES ABOUT 24
PREPARATION TIME: 15 minutes **COOKING TIME:** 12-15 minutes

Need a quick snack between meals? Then make up a batch of these delicious cookies, and keep them on hand to munch on.

1 cup apricots, chopped
⅓ cup boiling water
1 cup rolled oats
1 cup flour
½ cup oat bran
½ cup brown sugar
½ cup chopped walnuts
½ teaspoon baking powder
½ teaspoon each cinnamon and nutmeg
2 egg whites
¼ cup canola oil

♦ COVER the apricots with boiling water and let soak for 10 minutes. Cool.
♦ COMBINE the oats, sifted flour, oat bran, sugar, walnuts, baking powder, and spices in a large bowl.
♦ BEAT the egg whites until stiff, then add to cooled apricot mixture with the oil. Mix into dry ingredients.
♦ DROP tablespoonfuls of the mixture onto oiled baking trays, and bake at 350°F for 12–15 minutes, or until light brown. Let stand for 1 minute to cool before lifting off the tray. Store in an airtight container.

Nutrients per serving
Fat: 4.8 g, Saturated fat: 0.4 g, Fiber: 1.6 g, Sodium: 19 mg, Calories: 124,
Good for: soluble fiber, folate, antioxidants, low GI

❧ Five Things to Improve Your ❧ Diet Overnight

Fruit and Nut Snack Packs

MAKES ABOUT 5 CUPS (600 G) OR 10 SNACK PORTIONS
PREPARATION TIME: 10 minutes **COOKING TIME:** nil

Make these in bulk, and pack them into snack portions to nibble on during the day.

3 cups (13 oz) dried fruit medley (see Note)
1 cup (5 oz) dates
½ cup (3 oz) whole unpeeled almonds
½ cup (3 oz) walnut halves
4 tablespoons pepitas (pumpkin seeds)

❧ PLACE all ingredients in a large bowl. Toss to combine. Pack into 10 ziplock plastic bags or plastic containers.

NOTE
• Dried fruit medley is a mix of assorted fruit such as apricots, apples, raisins, pineapple chunks, and banana slices and is available at supermarkets. If you prefer, you can use 13 oz of any dried fruit you enjoy.

Nutrients per serving
Fat: 14.9 g, Saturated fat: 1.3 g, Fiber: 6.6 g, Sodium: 21 mg, Calories: 289,
Good for: soluble fiber, antioxidants, nuts, low GI

Linseed Sprinkle

MAKES ABOUT 1½ CUPS
PREPARATION TIME: 10 minutes **COOKING TIME:** nil

An easy way to take in more of the healthy fats, along with omega-3s, phytoestrogens, and fiber. Use this handy sprinkle over cereal, yogurt, fresh diced fruit, salads, and vegetables.

1 cup whole almonds or almond pieces
½ cup walnut pieces
½ cup linseeds

✦ PLACE almonds, walnuts, and linseeds in the bowl of a coffee grinder or food processor (you may have to do it in batches).
✦ PROCESS until finely ground. Store in a jar in the refrigerator to keep fresh. Use within a month.

Nutrients per serving
Fat: 8.3 g, Saturated fat: 0.6 g, Fiber: 2.2 g, Sodium: 2.0 mg, Calories: 92,
Good for: omega-3s, antioxidants, nuts, low GI

Baked Ricotta

> **MAKES 8 SERVEINGS**
> **PREPARATION TIME:** 10 minutes **COOKING TIME:** 30 minutes
> (unattended)

This baked ricotta can help you cut the fat in many ways—on toasted wood-fired bread instead of a high-fat cheese, with roasted vegetables or crackers as a pre-dinner nibble, or with fruit instead of cream. Because its flavor is neutral, it teams well with either savory or sweet foods. Make up a batch of it each week, store it in the refrigerator, and I guarantee you'll find it really handy.

1 lb fresh ricotta

➤ LINE a baking tray with wax paper. Pile the ricotta onto it. Using a flat knife, mold it into a round shape.

➤ BAKE at 350°F for 30 minutes, or until firm and just golden. The ricotta will "weep" a little moisture and flatten slightly during cooking. Cool, and store in refrigerator covered. Cut into wedges as needed.

VARIATION
- For a savory flavor to accompany vegetables or crusty bread, combine ricotta with 1 tablespoon finely chopped basil, 1 tablespoon finely chopped parsley, 1 teaspoon grated lemon rind, and freshly ground black pepper. Drizzle with 1 teaspoon olive oil, then bake.

NOTE
- If you want a more set shape, bake the ricotta in a pie plate or ovenproof dish. Press down hard with the back of a spoon to create a firm texture, and soak up any excess moisture with paper towels.

Nutrients per serving
Fat: 7.1 g, Saturated fat: 4.5 g, Fiber: 0 g, Sodium: 124 mg, Calories: 92

Super Smoothie

> **SERVES 1-2**
> **PREPARATION TIME:** 5 minutes **COOKING TIME:** nil

This smoothie gives you lots of nutrition for one-third of the fat and calories of normal milk shakes. And it's a delicious way to take in more oat bran for soluble fiber. Great for hungry teens and very active people.

1 cup low-fat milk or soy drink
1 ripe banana, sliced
1 tablespoon honey or sugar
¼ cup oat bran or rice bran
a few drops of vanilla essence (optional)

➤ PLACE all ingredients in a blender or food processor. Process for 30 seconds, or until blended and frothy.

VARIATION
- Instead of the banana, substitute ½ cup sliced strawberries or ½ cup fresh or frozen blueberries.

Nutrients per serving
Fat: 1.5 g, Saturated fat: 0.3 g, Fiber: 4.2 g, Sodium: 78 mg, Calories: 201, Good for: soluble fiber, soy protein, low GI

The Best Salad Dressing

MAKES ABOUT 1½ CUPS
PREPARATION TIME: 5 minutes **COOKING TIME:** nil

This is how to make salads and vegetables interesting! This dressing is easy to make, and it adds healthy fats to your meals. It keeps well in a bottle (refrigerate in warmer months).

1 cup extra-virgin olive oil
¼ cup balsamic vinegar
3–4 teaspoons Dijon mustard
2 cloves garlic, crushed
¼ teaspoon dried tarragon or basil
freshly ground black pepper

❥ PLACE all ingredients in a screwtop jar. Shake to combine well.

TIP
• For a lighter version, simply add 2 tablespoons water, and mix.

Nutrients per serving
Fat: 13.2 g, Saturated fat: 1.9 g, Fiber: 0.1 g, Sodium: 16 mg, Calories: 118,
Good for: antioxidants, low GI

More Help

WHERE TO GO FOR ADVICE AND INFORMATION

Professional advice

Your doctor
Your local doctor should be your first port of call for a simple blood test and coronary checkup. You can discuss your results and decide on any further testing or a referral to a specialist.

A cardiologist
If more help is needed, your doctor may refer you to a cardiologist who specializes in diagnosing and treating heart problems.

American Heart Association
The AHA is a national voluntary health agency whose mission is to reduce disability and death from cardiovascular disease. Formed in 1924, the AHA aims to alert people to the risk factors that cause heart disease. They run the very successful heart-checkmark food program. Items bearing the heart-check symbol are guaranteed to meet the AHA's standards for heart health.

Call toll-free 1-800-AHA-USA1 for printed materials about heart-healthy eating (including a copy of the AHA diet) and other heart-related topics.

American Stroke Association
A division of the AHA, the American Stroke Association offers a wide array of programs, products, and services to prevent and treat heart disease and stroke. Their storehouse of information

includes stroke risk factors and warning signs, life after stroke, and access to stroke support groups.

Call toll-free 1-888-4-STROKE for more information.

Consultation with a dietitian
Dietitians are experts on nutrition and can devise a personal eating plan to suit your particular needs or food preferences. To find a dietitian in your area, check the Yellow Pages. (Look for someone who is an RD, or registered dietitian).

American Dietetic Association
The ADA's mission is to promote optimal nutrition and well-being for all people. The ADA boasts nearly 70,000 food and nutrition professionals as members. Almost 75% of the members are registered dieticians.

ADA
216 W. Jackson Blvd.
Chicago, IL 60606-6995
312-899-0040
www.eatright.org

Web sites

www.americanheart.org
An extensive site from the American Heart Association dedicated to your heart. Has lots of useful information on risk factors, medical procedures, blood tests, alternatives to bypass surgery, the Ornish treatment, antioxidants, eggs, the Mediterranean Diet, cholesterol in children, and oat bran. Also gives the latest diet recommendations plus medical statements.

www.nhlbi.nih.gov/chd
An introduction to heart disease—what it is, what diet and medications to take—from the National Heart, Lung, and Blood Institute. The quizzes on cholesterol and heart disease IQ are

enlightening. Also, their Virtual Grocery Store and food label guide are excellent.

www.heartinfo.com
An educational site founded by a heart patient and a doctor, this has everything you want to know about heart troubles in a very accessible format. The best section is the latest news reports on heart research and treatment, but there's excellent material on heart-healthy cooking, a nutrition guide covering the latest diets, and a Lipids Newsletter.

www.foodwatch.com.au
If you want to stay up to date in nutrition, visit nutritionist Catherine Saxelby's web site, where you'll find recipes, quick quizzes, an A-to-Z nutrition dictionary, and summaries of food issues such as antioxidants, fats, vitamins, sterols, and folate. Updated regularly.

www.heartfoundation.com.au
This top Australian site covers a broad range of topics relating to heart problems, starting with general information and statistics on heart disease, through to research grants, material for schools and the media, and their food information program. There's a big emphasis on nutrition with topics like cholesterol, fat, alcohol, and low-fat cooking tips all given plenty of space. For doctors and dietitians, an excellent professional section covers key issues such as lipid-lowering drugs, plant sterols and stanols, omega-3s and fish oil, flaxseed oil, obesity, and vegetarian diets.

Recommended cookbooks

Many cookbooks today offer recipes and ideas for low-fat, healthy meals. Look for light, low-cholesterol, or low-fat cooking. Most books with traditional Italian, Greek, Spanish, or other Mediterranean recipes will be suitable. The same applies to Asian cookbooks.

The Complete Cooking Light Cookbook
Includes easy-to-follow, step-by-step instructions for more than 1,000 recipes. Also features lists of kitchen essentials for healthy eating. 528 pages. $34.95. Oxmoor House, 2000.

American Heart Association Low-Fat, Low-Cholesterol Cookbook
This fully revised edition presents a rich assortment of heart-healthy dishes from the AHA. Also includes plenty of tips on preparing foods more sensibly. 372 pages. $25.95. American Heart Association, 1998.

Everyday Cooking with Dean Ornish
The renowned cardiovascular researcher shares 150 extraordinary recipes that are all extremely low in fat and cholesterol. Slimmed-down versions of your favorite comfort foods. 368 pages. $15.95. HarperCollins, 1997.

Fresh & Healthy
The latest **Victor Chang Cardiac Research Institute Cookbook**
Another collaboration between Sally James and The Victor Chang Cardiac Research Institute, this book features 100 low-fat recipes (each superbly photographed), tips on alternative recipe substitutions, and a nutrition analysis. 160 pages. $34.95. ACP Publishing, 2000.

Glossary

Angiogram

A test that gives a picture of the arteries of the heart (a radiopaque dye is injected into the major arteries in the heart and picked up on a series of x-rays). It is used to diagnose heart disease and is essential before surgery.

Angioplasty (coronary angioplasty)

A surgical procedure that involves inserting a catheter with an inflatable balloon tip into a damaged artery in the heart. Starting at the skin, the catheter is threaded through the circulation, back toward the area of the heart where the diseased vessel is blocked. The balloon is then inflated against the blocked area to create a wide passage for blood flow. Introduced in the 1980s, it is less invasive than a bypass, as the chest does not have to be opened up, and it is done under local anesthetic.

Antioxidant

Any substance that prevents or delays damage of cells or genetic material by free radicals such as reactive oxygen and reactive nitrogen compounds. Vegetables, fruits, nuts, and oil seeds are high in the antioxidant vitamins C and E and beta-carotene. Phytochemicals found in foods, such as the catechins in tea or the phenols in wine, also act as antioxidants.

Arrhythmia

Abnormal or irregular rhythm of the heart that can be responsible for sudden, fatal heart attacks.

Arteriosclerosis

Often referred to as "hardening of the arteries." Refers to any of a number of changes that lead to thickening, loss of elasticity, and hardening of the walls of the arteries, which eventually narrows or stops the flow of blood.

Atherosclerosis

Thickening and clogging of the large arteries due to an accumulation of fat, cholesterol, calcium, and other material on the inside walls, which is the underlying process of heart disease. This thickening can narrow and obstruct the arteries, reducing or cutting off the flow of blood to the heart (which causes heart attack, angina, or sudden death) or to the brain (which causes a stroke). The most common form of arteriosclerosis.

Cardiovascular disease

An all-encompassing term used to describe all diseases and conditions involving the heart and blood vessels (arteries or veins), including coronary heart disease, stroke, peripheral heart disease, and heart failure. The main underlying problem in heart disease is atherosclerosis (see above).

Cholesterol

A white, tasteless, fat-like substance normally present in the blood, which plays an important role in many bodily functions such as producing hormones, insulating nerve fibers, and forming bile acids. A high level of blood cholesterol is one of the risk factors for heart disease.

Coronary heart disease

Any disorder of the heart or blood vessels (arteries or veins) that affects the supply of blood specifically to the heart.

Fatty acids

Building blocks of fat molecules. They can be saturated, monounsaturated, or polyunsaturated.

HDL cholesterol

High-density lipoprotein cholesterol. Also known as the "good" cholesterol, as it has a protective effect against heart disease.

Infarct

Short for myocardial infarction, the medical term for a heart attack caused by the "death" of a heart muscle when it is starved of oxygen due to a blocked artery.

Ischemic heart disease

Another term for heart disease.

LDL cholesterol

Low-density lipoprotein cholesterol. Also known as the "bad" cholesterol, as high levels in the blood can stick to artery walls, causing a blockage.

Lipids

General term embracing all fats, oils, and waxy substances that are insoluble in water. In medical jargon, blood lipids refer to triglycerides and cholesterol—both free and when bound to lipoprotein (HDL and LDL cholesterol).

Lipoprotein

Particles of liquid (fat) that are coated with protein to enable the lipid to be transported in the bloodstream.

Monosaturated

Refers to the bonds in a carbon chain of a fatty acid. There is one bond between individual carbon atoms, and this is a double bond, e.g., oleic acid. Foods with a high content of monounsaturated fatty acids include olive oil, canola oil, canola margarines, most nuts, and avocados.

Omega-3s

Types of polyunsaturated fatty acids such as EPA and DHA, found in fish, as well as lineolic acid in flaxseed and canola.

Omega-6s

Types of polyunsaturated fatty acids, such as linoleic acid, which are the main components of common oils (sunflower, safflower, maize, cottonseed) and polyunsaturated margarines. Our current diet is presently skewed towards omega-6s and should be closer to the ideal ratio of 5–6 parts omega-6 to one part of omega-3.

Plasma lipids

Blood fats such as cholesterol and triglycerides.

Polyunsaturated

Refers to the bonds in a carbon chain of a fatty acid. Polyunsaturated fatty acids have two or more bonds between individual carbon atoms, e.g., linoleic acid, gamma-linoleic acid. Can be further classified into omega-3 and omega-6 fatty acids. Foods with a high content of polyunsaturated fatty acids include safflower oil, sunflower oil, polyunsaturated margarines, walnuts, wheat germ, and most seeds.

Saturated

Refers to the bonds in a carbon chain of a fatty acid. The bonds between individual carbon atoms of a saturated fat hold as many hydrogen atoms as possible, e.g., stearic acid, palmitic acid. Foods with a high content of saturated fatty acids include butter, cream, fat on meat, coconut oil, and palm oil.

Serum lipids

Blood fats such as cholesterol and triglycerides.

Stenting (coronary stenting)

A surgical procedure similar to angioplasty that involves inserting an expandable metal mesh-like tube within the major artery of the heart to support and hold the artery open at the point where there is narrowing.

Triglycerides

A form of fat in food and the body consisting of glycerol plus three fatty acids. A high level of blood triglycerides is a risk factor for heart disease and stroke and is usually raised by being overweight and by excess alcohol.

References

General

British Cardiac Society et al. "Joint British recommendations on prevention of coronary heart disease in clinical practice: summary." Br Med J 2000; 320: 705–8.

Grundy, S.M., Pasternak, R., Greenland, P. et al. "AHA/ACC Scientific Statement. Assessment of cardivascular risk by use of multiple-risk-factor assessment equations." Circulation 1999; 100: 1481–92.

Jackson, R. "Guidelines on preventing cardiovascular disease in clinical practice." Br Med J 2000; 320: 659–61.

Noakes, M., Clifton, P., McMurchie, T. "Diet can make a difference. Review of the functions of foods in improving heart and digestive health." Aust J Nutr & Dietetics 1999; 56: 3 S1–S34.

Stampfer, M.J., Hu, F.B., Manson, J.E. et al. "Primary prevention of coronary heart disease in women through diet and lifestyle." N Engl J Med 2000; 343: 16–22.

Studies of particular dietary patterns

Appel, L.J., Moore, T.J., Obarzanek, E. et al. "A clinical trial of the effects of dietary patterns on blood pressure." N Engl J Med 1997; 336: 1117–24.

Burr, M.L., Gilbert, J.F., Holliday, R.M. et al. "Effects of changes in fat, fish and fibre intakes on death and myocardial reinfarction: Diet and Reinfarction Trial (DART)." Lancet 1989; 757–61.

De Lorgeril, M., Salen, P., Martin, J.L. "Mediterranean diet, traditional risk factors, and the rate of cardiovascular complications after myocardial infarction: Final report of the Lyon Diet Heart Study." Circulation 1999: 99; 779–85.

References

Studies on fish and omega-3s

Connor, S.L., Connor, W.E. "Are fish oils beneficial in the prevention and treatment of coronary artery disease?" Am J Clin Nutr 1997; 66 (suppl): 1020S–31S.

De Deckere, E.A.M., Korver, O., Verschuren, P.M. et al. "Health aspects of fish and n-3 polyunsaturated fatty acids from plant and marine origin." Eur J Clin Nutr 1998; 52: 749–53.

Harris, W.S., "N-3 fatty acids and serum lipoproteins: human studies." Am J Clin Nutr 1997; 65(suppl): 1645S–54S.

Knapp, H.R. "Dietary fatty acids in human thrombosis and hemostasis." Am J Clin Nutr 1997; 65 (suppl): 1687S–98S.

Roche, H.M., Gibney, M.J. "Effect of long-chain n-3 polyunsaturated fatty acids on fasting and postpriandial triacylglycerol metabolism." Am J Clin Nutr 2000; 71 (suppl): 232S–7S. [This is one of 38 papers in an entire supplement of this journal devoted to omega-3 fats and well worth reading. There are 6 papers specifically covering omega-3s and heart disease.]

Stark, K.D., Park, E.J., Maines, V.A. et al. "Effect of a fish-oil concentrate on serum lipids in postmenopausal women receiving and not receiving hormone replacement therapy in a placebo-controlled double blind trial." Am J Clin Nutr 2000; 72: 389–94.

Von Shacky, C., Angerer, P., Kothny, W. et al. "The effect of dietary n-3 fatty acids on coronary atherosclerosis. A randomised double-blind placebo-controlled trial." Ann Intern Med 1999; 130: 554–62.

Weber, P., Raederstorff, D. "Triglyceride-lowering effect of omega-3 LC-polyunsaturated fatty acids – a review." Nutr Metab Cardiovasc Dis 2000; 10: 28–37.

Studies on sterols

Gylling, H., Miettinen, T.A. "Effects of inhibiting cholesterol absorption and synthesis on cholesterol and lipoprotein metabolism in hypercholesterolemic non-insulin dependent diabetic men." J Lipid Res 1996; 37(8): 1776–85.

Gylling, H., Radharkrishnan, R., Miettinen, T.A. "Reduction of serum cholesterol in postmenopausal women with previous myocardial

References

infarction and cholesterol malabsorption induced by dietary sitostanol-ester margarine. Women and dietary sitostanol." Circulation 1997; 96: 422–31.

Hallikainen, M.A., Uusitupa, M.I.J. "Effects of 2 low-fat stanol ester-containing margarines on serum cholesterol part of a low-fat diet in hypercholesterolemic subjects." Am J Clin Nutr 1999; 69: 403–10.

Heart Foundation's Nutrition and Metabolism Advisory Committee. Plant sterols and stanols Position Statement 1999.

Miettinen, T.A., Puska, P., Gylling, H. et al "Reduction of serum cholesterol with sitostanol-ester margarine in a mildly hypercholesterolaemic population." N Engl J Med 1995; 333: 1308–12.

Normen, L., Dutta, P., Lia, A. et al. "Soy sterol esters and beta-sitosterol ester as inhibitors of cholesterol absorption in the human small bowel." Am J Clin Nutr 2000; 71(4): 908–13.

Simons, L.A. "Diet and blood cholesterol. Role of plant sterol-enriched spreads." Current Therapeutics October 1999: 40(10); 11–13.

Westrate, J.A., Meijer, G.W. "Plant-sterol enriched margarines and reduction of plasma total and LDL cholesterol concentrations in normocholesterolaemic and mildly hypercholesterolaemic subjects." Eur J Clin Nutr 1998; 52: 334–43.

Studies on antioxidants/fruit and vegetables

Klipstein-Grobusch, K., Geleijnse, J.M., den Breeijan, J.H. et al. "Dietary antioxidants and risk of myocardial infarction in the elderly: the Rotterdam Study." Am J Clin Nutr 1999; 69: 261–6.

Kushi, L.H., Folsom, A.R., Prineas, R.J. et al. "Dietary antioxidant vitamins and death from coronary heart disease in postmenopausal women." N Engl J Med 1996; 334: 1156–62.

Kushi, L.H., Lenart, E.B., Willet, W.C. "Health implications of Mediterranean diets in light of contemporary knowledge. 1. Plant foods and dairy products." Am J Clin Nutr 1995; 61 Suppl: 1407–15.

Joshipura, K., Ascherios, A., Manson, J. et al. "Fruit and vegetable intake in relation to risk of ischaemic stroke." JAMA 1999; 282: 1233–9.

References

Liu, S., Manson, J.E., Lee, I-M. et al. "Fruit and vegetable intake and risk of cardiovascular disease: the Women's Health Study." Am J Clin Nutr 2000; 72: 922–8.

Rimm, E.B., Ascherio, A., Giovanucci, E. at al. "Vegetable, fruit and cereal fibre intake and risk of coronary heart disease among men." JAMA 1996; 275: 447–51.

Yochum, L.A., Folsom, A.R., Kushi, L.H. "Intake of antioxidant vitamins and risk of death from stroke in postmenopausal women." Am J Clin Nutr 2000; 72: 476–83.

Studies on tea

Geleijnse, J.M., Launer, L.J., Hofman, A. et al. "Tea flavonoids protect against atherosclerosis. The Rotterdam Study." Arch Intern Med 1999; 159(18): 2170–4.

Hertog, M.G.L., Feskens, E.K.M., Hollman, P.C.H. et al. "Dietary anti-oxidant flavonoids and risk of coronary heart disease: The Zutphen Elderly Study." Lancet 1993; 342: 1007–11.

Keli, S.O., Hertog, M.G.L., Feskens, E.J.M. et al. "Dietary flavonoids, antioxidant vitamins and incidence of stroke." Arch Intern Med 1996; 154: 637–42.

Sesso, H.D., Gaziano, J.M., Buring, J.E. et al. "Coffee and tea intake and the risk of myocardial infarction." Am J Epidemiol 1999; 149 (2): 162–7.

Studies on whole grains and glycaemic index

Frost, G., Leeds, A.A., Dore, C.J. et al. "Gycaemic index as a determinant of serum HDL-cholesterol concentration." Lancet 1999; 2353: 1045–8.

Jacobs, D.R., Meyer, K.A., Kushi, L.H. et al. "Whole grain intake may reduce the risk of ischemic heart disease death in postmenopausal women: The Iowa Women's Health Study." Am J Clin Nutr 1998; 68: 248–57.

Liu, S., Stampfer, M.J., Hu, F.B. et al. "Whole-grain consumption and risk of coronary heart disease: results from the Nurses' Health Study." Am J Clin Nutr 1999; 70: 412–9.

Liu, S., Willet, W.C., Stampfer, M.J. et al. "A prospective study of

References

dietary glycaemic load, carbohydrate intake and risk of coronary heart disease in US women." Am J Clin Nutr 2000; 71: 1455–61.

Slavin, J.L., Martini, M.C., Jacobs, D.R. et al. "Plausible mechanisms for the protectiveness of whole grains." Am J Clin Nutr 1999; 70(suppl): 459S–63S.

Truswell, A.S. Cereal grains and coronary heart disease: a review of the literature. Grains Res and Dev Corporation and BRI Australia Ltd, 2000.

Studies on soy protein

The role of soy in preventing and treating chronic disease. Am J Clin Nutr 1999; 68: 1329S–1544S.

Anderson, J.W. "Meta-analysis of the effects of soy protein intake on serum lipids." N Engl J Med 1995; 333: 276–82.

Merz-Demlow, B., Duncan, A., Wangen, K. et al. "Soy isoflavones improve plasma lipids in normocholesterolemic, premenopausal women." Am J Clin Nutr 2000; 71: 1461–9.

Washburn, S., Burke, G.L., Morgan, T. et al. "Effect of soy protein supplementation on serum lipoproteins, blood pressure and menopausal symptoms in perimenopausal women." Menopause 1990; 6: 7–13.

Studies on nuts

Abbey, M., Noakes, M., Belling, G.B. et al. "Partial replacement of saturated fatty acids with almonds or walnuts lowers total plasma cholesterol and low-density-lipoprotein cholesterol." Am J Clin Nutr 1994; 59: 995–9.

Curb, J.D., Wergowske, G., Dobbs, J.C. et al. "Serum lipid effects of a high-monounsaturated fat diet based on macadamia nuts." Arch Intern Med 2000; 160: 1154–8.

Hu, F.B., Stampfer, M.J., Manson, J.E. at al. "Frequent nut consumption and risk of coronary heart disease in women: prospective cohort study." (Breakout) Med J 1998; 713: 1341–5.

Kris-etherton, P.M., Yu-Poth, S., Sabate, J. et al. "Nuts and their bioactive constitutents: effects on serum lipids and other factors that affect disease risk." Am J Clin Nutr 1999; 70 Suppl: 540S–51S.

References

Sabate, J. "Nut consumption, vegetarian diets, ischaemic heart disease risk, and all-cause mortality: evidence from epidemiological studies." Am J Clin Nutr 1999; 70 Suppl: 500S–03S.

Zambon, D., Sabate, J., Munoz, S. et al. "Substituting walnuts for monounsaturated fat improves the serum lipid profile of hypercholesterolamic men and women." Ann Intern Med 2000; 132: 538–46.

Studies on soluble fiber

Anderson, J., Allgood, L., Lawrence, A. et al. "Cholesterol-lowering effects of psyllium intake adjective to diet therapy in men and women with hyperchol-esterolemia:meta-analysis of 8 controlled trials." Am J Clin Nutr 2000; 71: 472–9.

Anderson, J., Davidson, M., Blonde, L. et al. "Long-term cholesterol lowering effect of psyllium as an adjunct to diet therapy in the treatment of hypercholesterolemia." Am J Clin Nutr 2000; 71: 1433–8.

Brown, I., Rosner, B., Willett, W.W. "Cholesterol-lowering effects of dietary fibre: a meta-analysis." Am J Clin Nutr 1999; 69: 30–42.

Glore, S.R., Van Treeck, D., Knehans, A.W. et al. "Soluble fibre and serum lipids: a literature review." J Am Diet Assoc 1994; 94(4): 425–36.

Leeds, A.R. "Psyllium – a superior source of soluble dietary fibre." Food Aust 1995; 42, 2:S1–4.

Olson, B.H., Anderson, S.M., Becker, M.P. et al. "Psyllium-enriched cereals lower blood total cholesterol and LDL cholesterol, but not HDL cholesterol, in hypercholesterolamic adults: results of a meta-analysis." J Nutr 1997; 127: 1973–80.

Rispin, C.M. et al. "Oat products and lipid-lowering: a meta-analysis." JAMA 1992; 267: 3317–25.

Studies on folate and homocysteine

"Homocysteine, diet and cardiovascular diseases." Circulation AHA, 1999 March 17; 99: 178–83.

Grubben, M.J., Boers, G.H., Blom, H.J. et al. "Unfiltered coffee increases plasma homocysteine concentrations in healthy volunteers: a randomised trial." Am J Clin Nutr 2000; 71: 480–4.

References

Homocysteine Lowering Trialists' Collab-oration. "Lowering blood homocysteine with folic acid based supplements: meta-analysis of randomised trials." BMJ 1998; 316 (7135): 894–8.

Riddell, L., Chisholm, A., Williams, S. et al. "Dietary strategies for lowering homocysteine concentrations." Am J Clin Nutr 2000; 71: 1448–54.

Studies on garlic

Adler, A.J., Holub, B.J. "Effect of garlic and fish oil suplementation on serus lipid and lipoprotein concentrations in hypercholesterolemic men." Am J Clin Nutr 1997; 65: 445–50.

Steiner, M., Hakim Khan, A., Holbert, D. et al. "A double-blind crossover study in moderately hypercholesterolemic men that compared the effect of aged garlic extract and placebo administration on blood lipids." Am J Clin Nutr 1996; 64: 866–70.

Stevinson, C., Pittler, M.H., Ernst, E. "Garlic for treating hypercholesterolemia: a meta-analysis of randomised clinical trials." Ann Intern Med 2000; 133: 420–9.

Studies on alcohol

Cuevas, A.M., Guash, V., Castillo, O. "A high-fat diet induces, and red wine counteracts, endothelial dysfunction in human volunteers." Lipids 2000; 35 (2): 143–8.

Gronbaek, M., Deis, A., Sorensen, T.I.A. et al. "Mortality associated with moderate intake of wines, beers and spirits." Br Med J 1995; 310: 1165–9.

Klatsky, A.L., Armstrong, M.A. "Alcoholic beverage choice and risk of coronary heart disease mortality: do red wine drinkers fare best?" Am J Cardiol 1993; 71: 467–9.

Krankel, E.N., Kanner, J., German, J.B. et al. "Inhibition of oxidation of human low-density lipoprotein by phenolic substances in red wine." Lancet 1993; 341: 454–7.

Yang, T., Doherty, T., Wong, N. et al. "Alcohol consumption, coronary calcium, and coronary heart disease events." Am J Cardiol 1999; 84: 802–06.

References

Studies on vitamin E

GISSI-Prevenzione Investigators. "Dietary supplementation with n-3 polyunsaturated fatty acids and vitamin E after myocardial infarction: results of the GISSI-Prevenzione trial." Lancet 1999; 354: 447–55.

The Heart Outcomes Prevention Evaluation Study Investigators. "Vitamin E supplementation and cardiovascular events in high-risk patients." N Engl J Med 2000; 342(3): 154–60.

Mottram, P., Shige, H., Nestel, P. "Vitamin E improves arterial compliance in middle-aged men and women." Atherosclerosis 1999; 145: 399–404.

Porkkala-Srartaho, E.K., Nyyssonen, M.K., Kaikkonen, J.E. et al. "A randomised single-blind placebo-controlled trial of the effects of 200 mg alpha-tocopherol on the oxidation resistance of atherogenic lipoproteins." Am J Clin Nutr 1998; 68: 1034–41.

Simons, L.A., Von Konigsmark, M., Balasubramaniam, S. "What dose of vitamin E is required to reduce susceptibility of LDL to oxidation." Aust N Z J Med 1996; 26: 496–502.

Stephens, N.G., Parsons, A., Scholfield, P.M. et al. "Randomised controlled trial of vitamin E in patients with coronary heart disease: Cambridge Heart Antioxidant Study (CHAOS)." Lancet 1996; 347: 781–6.

Others

Grubben, M.J., Boers, G.H., Blom, H.J. et al. "Unfiltered coffee increases plasma homocysteine concentrations in healthy volunteers: a randomised trial." Am J Clin Nutr 2000; 71: 480–4.

Heber, D., Yip, I., Ashley, J. et al. "Cholesterol-lowering effects of a proprietary Chinese red-yeast-rice dietary supplement." AJCN 1999; 69: 231–6.

Noakes, M., Nestel, P.J., Clifton, P.M. "Commercial frying fats and plasma lipid-lowering potential." Aust J Nutr Diet 1996; 53: 25–30.

Urgert, R., van Vliet, T., Zock, P.L. et al. "Heavy coffee consumption and plasma homocysteine: a randomised controlled tiral in healthy volunteers." Am J Clin Nutr 200; 72: 1107–10.

Index

Page numbers in *italics* refer to glossary terms.
The Recipe Index follows the General Index.

A

abdomen, excess weight on, 24–25
advice, professional, 195–196
alcohol, effect on the heart, 91–92
    studies on, 210
angiogram, *201*
angioplasty (coronary angioplasty), *201*
antioxidants, *201*
    chart describing role in recipes, 126
    foods rich in, 42–44, 45–46
    function in body, 41–43
    studies on, 206
arginine, nuts and, 49
arrythmia (irregular heartbeat), *201*
arteriosclerosis, *201–202*
    definition of, *xv*
Asian food
    menu ideas, 82–83 (*see also Recipe Index*)
    ordering healthy, 98–99
aspirin, effect on heart disease, 107–108
associations, heart
    American Dietetic Association, 196
    American Heart Association (AHA), 195
    American Stroke Association, 196
atherosclerosis, *202*
    definition of, *xv*

B

"bad" cholesterol. *see* LDL cholesterol
"baked not fried," foods labeled as, 72–73

baked potatoes, ordering healthy, 98
beans, types to stock up on, 63
beer, effect on the heart, 91–92
bile acid resins, effect on heart disease, 106–107
black tea. *see* tea
blood pressure
    high, and heart disease, 12–13
    lowering, tips on, 94
    normal, range considered, 13
body fat
    menu suggestions to lose, 78–79
    shedding excess, 23, 24–25
breads, types to stock up on, 64
breakfast, menu ideas. *see also Recipe Index*
    Asian style, 83
    cereals, types to stock up on, 65
    to lose body fat, 78
    to maintain current weight, 79
    Mediterranean-style, 80
    on-the-go, 84–85
    vegetarian, 81–82
burritos, ordering healthy, 98
butter, alternatives to, 60

C

caffeine, effect on the heart, 92–93
calories
    recommended daily amount of, 125
cardiovascular disease, *202*
cereals, types to stock up on, 65
cheese
    cooking with, 76
    types to stock up on, 67
chicken
    choosing low-fat, 100
chicken, ordering healthy, 97
Chinese food, ordering healthy, 98

Index

Index

Index

Index

Index

Vietnamese food, ordering healthy, 98
visible fats, 99–100
vitamin E
    nuts and, 49
    studies on, 211
    as supplement, 108–109

W

web sites, recommended, 196–198
weight
    and heart disease, 24–25

menu ideas to maintain current, 79–80
whole grains
    benefits to body, 51–52
    chart describing role in recipes, 126
    studies on, 207
    ways to include in diet, 53
wine, effect on the heart, 91–92
wraps, ordering healthy, 98

Y

yogurts, types to stock up on, 67

Recipe Index

Recipe Index

Recipe Index

Recipe Index